Sex Pos for Couples

The Ultimate Sex Book
for Couples with Kama Sutra and
Tantric Techniques for Beginners
and Advanced.

Riley Ashwood

Table of Contents

CONCLUSION   137

Introduction

Welcome to *Sex Positions for Couples,* and thank you for Purchasing. In this book, I will take you on a journey of exploration. Read this book with an open mind, and you will learn a myriad of ways to take your sex life to the next level as a couple. Through reading this book, you will learn new techniques and skills like new sex positions and how best to lead a woman to orgasm. You will also learn other types of skills such as how to increase intimacy and how to get into the mood. This book touches on every aspect of sex from beginning to end and will allow you to hone your sex skills in order to impress your partner and strengthen your relationship. If you have ever wondered what else you can do to improve your sex life, or what might be missing, this book will show you all of that and more. By reading this book, even the sections that you may think you know already, you will be able to brush up on things you are familiar with, which is always a good thing.

There are some things to keep in mind when it comes to sex, and in this introduction, we will cover these first before diving in. The first thing we are going to discuss are the differences to keep in mind when having sex in a relationship versus casual sex. For some of you, relationship sex may be new, or it may be a while since you have been in a relationship. For this reason, we are going to go over some things that you should note when you enter a relationship. Communication is the key to a good relationship, sex aside. When it comes to sex, communication is key there, as well. This is especially true when in a long-term relationship. When having casual sex, communication is helpful since then you can figure out what the person likes and dislikes, but oftentimes it takes trial and error to find out how to please that person. Likely by the time you figure out exactly how to do so, you have moved onto the next person. When having sex in a relationship, you have much more time to talk about sex and find out what that person likes and dislikes. You may even feel more pressure to please them since you value their feelings and want to make them feel good. Being able to communicate during sex is great for a relationship because you can be learning in the moment. When you are learning in the moment, you know exactly what the person is referring to instead of having to recall it later. This does not have to happen like a visit to the doctor where they ask you "does this hurt?" you can indicate to each other what you like by telling them that "this feels good" or "keep going" without ruining the sensual mood. Being able to do this will help both of you to be pleased in the long-term.

The other reason that communication is so essential in a relationship sex is that people's likes and needs change over time. If you have been with someone for six years, they may have developed new preferences in terms of their pleasure. Being able to communicate this will allow for continued pleasure no matter how long you are together. Aside from changing needs, you and your partner want to keep sex interesting. When you are having casual sex, you will meet up once or twice and do whatever feels good that day. When you are in a relationship, you will likely develop somewhat of a routine that you know gives you both pleasure every time. This can become dull after a while, so being able to communicate about what you both would like to try will help to keep your sex life new and fresh. It is rare that you will talk about sex and new things that you would like to try in the bedroom with a one-night stand, but when in a relationship having talks about sex outside of the bedroom in times when you aren't horny will keep you both informed about where the other person stands when it comes to sex.

By taking the above into consideration, you will be well on your way to having a fulfilling and pleasurable sex life no matter how long you have been in a relationship for. A dull sex life is not inevitable, and by maintaining the lines of communication in your relationship, you will be able to keep yourselves happy and fulfilled. In addition to being fulfilled sexually, this will keep you both fulfilled in your relationship as a whole. A good sex life is important to having a close and healthy relationship. Prioritizing this will lead to a better overall relationship. Sex is hard to talk about, so being able to do this will strengthen your bond overall.

One final tip on this topic is to be open-minded when discussing these things with your partner. It may be hard for them to open up to you about things that they want to try or how they want you to please them. Being open-minded and non-judgmental will help them to feel safe and secure in this territory. This goes for all genders. Men will often not voice their insecurities when it comes to sex, but this does not mean they don't have them. By being open and listening to their desires, they will feel safe opening up to you over and over again. Getting comfortable with these types of dialogues can take time, so have patience with yourself and your partner, and most of all, enjoy!

In the rest of this book, we will delve into more specific sex topics. All focused on improving your long-term relationship sex life. Read on for more.

Chapter 1
Intimacy

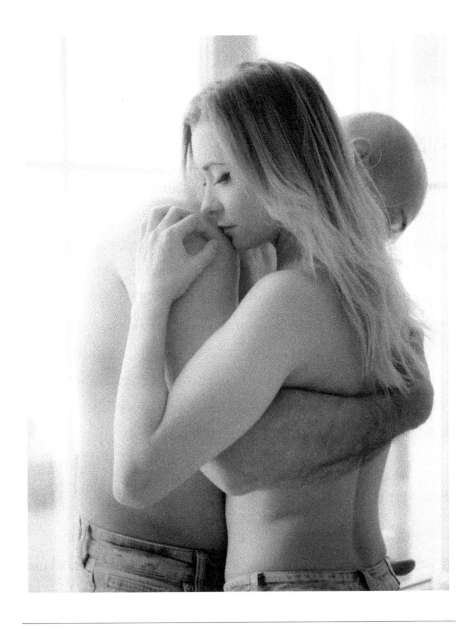

We will begin this book by discussing intimacy. Intimacy is very important between two people when part of a couple, especially in the bedroom. Intimacy is what brings you close and keeps you close. For this reason, we are going to address intimacy in this first chapter before moving onto sex positions and techniques for couples. Firstly, we will look at what intimacy means and the different types of intimacy that exist.

What Is Intimacy

There are different types of intimacy, and here I will outline them for you before digging deeper into intimacy for couples. Intimacy, in a general sense, is defined as mutual openness and vulnerability. There are different ways in which you can give and receive openness and vulnerability. Intimacy does not have to include a sexual relationship (though it can). Therefore, it is not only reserved for romantic relationships. Intimacy can also be present in other types of close relationships like friendships or family relationships. Below, I will outline the different forms of intimacy.

Emotional

Emotional intimacy is the ability to express oneself in a mature and open manner, leading to a deep emotional connection between people. Saying things like "I love you" or "you are very important to me" are examples of this. It is also the ability to respond in a mature and open way when someone expresses themselves to you by saying things like "I'm sorry" or "I love you too."

Intellectual

Intellectual intimacy is a kind of intimacy that involves discussing and sharing thoughts and opinions on intellectual matters, from which they gain fulfillment and feelings of closeness with the other person. For example, if you are discussing politics with someone who you deem to be an intellectual equal, you may find that you feel a closeness with them as you share your thoughts and opinions and connect on an intellectual level. Many people find intellect and brains to be sexy in a partner!

Shared Interests and Activities

This form of intimacy is less well-known, but it is also considered a form of intimacy. When you share activities with another person that you both enjoy and are passionate about, this creates a sense of connection. For example, when you cook together or travel together. These shared experiences give you memories to share, and this leads to bonding and intimacy (openness and vulnerability).

Physical

Physical intimacy is the type that most people think of when they hear the term, and it is the kind that we will be most concerned within this book, as it is the type of intimacy that includes sex and all activities related to sex. It also involves other non-sexual types of physical contact such as hugging and kissing. Physical intimacy can be found in close friendships or familial relationships where hugging and kisses on the cheek are common.

How to Improve Intimacy

For a romantic relationship to be successful, there must be several forms of intimacy shared between the partners. Without intimacy, there is nothing that sets a romantic relationship apart from an everyday friendship.

Determine Compatibility

In romantic relationships, every person will value different forms of intimacy over others or have certain forms of intimacy that are non-negotiable in terms of being included in a relationship for them. Your compatibility with a person will be largely dependent on which forms of intimacy you deem necessary and which you can live without, and how these preferences work together.

In order to determine your romantic compatibility with someone, use the following tool. Each of you will rate each of the four forms of intimacy as a 1, 2, or 3. A rating of 1 means that it is absolutely necessary, a rating of 2 means that it is somewhat necessary but not a deal-breaker and a rating of 3 means that it is unimportant to you. After each of your rates all four types of intimacy, you will compare your ratings. To determine compatibility from these results, you will look at which of your ratings are the same and which of them are opposites (1 and 3). If you have mostly the same scores or a 1 and a 2 for example, you are compatible with this person. If you mostly rated opposites (1 and 3), then you are likely incompatible with a romantic relationship with this person. While there are other factors to take into account when determining compatibility with someone, this measure focuses only on compatibility for intimacy. It is ultimately up to you to decide if you feel you are compatible with someone.

If there are several points where there are number two's, this can be a point of conversation for the two of you. You can discuss what makes that specific type of intimacy a number 2 and not a 1 or a 3. This will give you insight into the person's thoughts, and this activity alone can be a way to improve intimacy as you will need to be open and vulnerable with each other.

If you determine that you are compatible with the person but that the intimacy is lacking in your relationship, there are ways that it can be developed and improved. Further, if there are certain forms of intimacy that are lacking or if intimacy, in general, is lacking in a relationship where it once was, there are ways that this can be improved as well.

Communication

The first way to restore intimacy in a relationship or to develop it in the first place is through communication. Communication is key in a relationship of any sort, but especially in a romantic relationship. Communicating is the only sure way to know where the other person stands in terms of their thoughts and feelings. Being able to be vulnerable and open with your emotions is a requirement for intimacy. It is necessary to share oneself with the other person in a relationship. This mutual sharing of yourselves is what will lead to intimacy in the first place or an increase in intimacy.

Sometimes in a long-term relationship, you become so comfortable with each other that you don't have to communicate as much as you used to since you know each other so well. The key here is to continue communicating, even if you think the other person knows what you are thinking or feeling without you having to say it. By doing this, you keep the lines of communication open in your relationship. This avoids any chance of miscommunication or misunderstanding that would be perpetuated by a lack of communication. By having misunderstandings go unresolved, this could lead to resentment and an overall breakdown in communication, which can reduce levels of intimacy in the relationship.

Returning to the activity that I mentioned earlier about determining compatibility and discussing your answers with your partner, this is a great way for people who are already in a relationship to learn about the intimacy requirements of their partner. If your partner doesn't care whether you have shared activities or not, for example, ask them more about this to learn why this is. You will likely find out some new things about them and how they prefer to connect with you. Maybe they simply value emotional and intellectual intimacy over shared activities. Take turns sharing your reasoning and your feelings about the different forms of intimacy and how they rank in your mind. This type of communication allows you to address the topic of intimacy and this dialogue will be helpful in improving the intimacy in your relationship.

By learning these things about your partner, you can begin to work together to ensure each person's intimacy needs are met. For example, if your number one intimacy preference is for emotional intimacy and your partner likes to show their love in physical ways, you can discuss how they can begin to be more vocal about their love for you, and you can be more receptive to their physical displays of affection. Putting these things out on the table for discussion is the best way to learn about each other. You can never stop learning about your partner, and this will only strengthen your relationship.

It is important to communicate about your needs for intimacy on a recurring basis since people will grow and change over the course of a relationship. Especially in a long-term relationship, being aware of when a person's intimacy needs change is important to maintaining a good level of intimacy.

Start Slowly

Whether you are at the beginning of your relationship or trying to restore intimacy where it once was, it can be hard to jump right to the deepest topics of conversation like your dating history or your childhood. When working on intimacy, it is helpful to start slow by talking about things that are easier for you to open up about- like your future goals or your ideal job. This is still a way to open up without pushing yourself too far right away. It can be scary to be that vulnerable with someone. It is also helpful to note that for many people, there are things that they consciously avoid thinking about, as they may be painful to address. It will be very difficult for them to voice these things to themselves, let alone another person, so allow them to start slowly and don't be offended if you feel like there are topics that they are uncomfortable talking about.

Patience

When it comes to a newer relationship, it can be difficult to determine if you are at a comfortable level of intimacy, since you are still getting to know the person on a deeper and deeper level. Intimacy requires patience at the beginning of a relationship since it takes work to build it over time. If your relationship is in the newer stages, be patient when it comes to intimacy as the person you are with may still be getting comfortable opening up to you, or they may not be quite comfortable being vulnerable yet. By being aware of this, you can continue to open the lines of communication more and more, and over time this will lead to an increase in intimacy. In the beginning, you may have more physical intimacy and less emotional intimacy but with time and as your relationship develops, you will be able to improve your level of intimacy.

Many people have a fear of intimacy, and this is also worth noting. Because intimacy needs trust in order to develop, it can be hard for some people who have had past experiences that make it hard for them to trust people. By being aware of this, it may help you to understand why your partner has trouble opening up. It may also help you if you have a fear of intimacy as you can explain this to your partner in order to ask for the patience you will need as you begin to open up and be vulnerable with them.

When it comes to improving intimacy, it is a slow build and not a race to the finish line. Be patient with yourself and your partner, and try to see intimacy as a growing experience between you that will continue throughout the entire duration of your relationship.

Chapter 2
The Kama Sutra

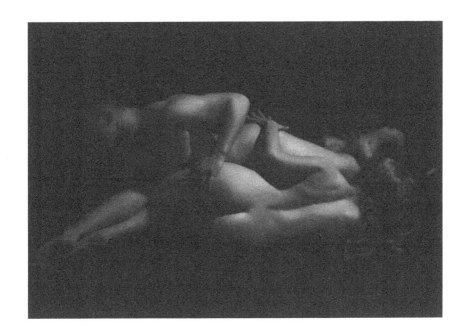

Following the previous chapter on intimacy, in this chapter, we will discuss The Kama Sutra. You may have heard this before in discussions of sex positions and experimental sex acts, but in reality, The Kama Sutra is much more than this. We will examine its history and how it relates to relationship sex in more detail below.

What Is the Kama Sutra?

The Kama Sutra is a guide book for love and everything involved in loving another person. It is more than just a book of sex positions, but these days most people only know it for its complex and flexibility-requiring positions for intercourse. The book of Kamasutra includes a general guide to living well in ways other than through sex. It includes a guide to foreplay, a guide to kissing and touching, as well as other ways to achieve intimacy with your partner, such as bathing together and giving each other massages.

It does include the sex positions it is most known for, as well as guides and positions for other types of sex, including oral sex and masturbation. The Kamasutra also touches on same-sex relationships, calling this the *third nature*. It also touches on group relations and a little bit of rough sex. The Kamasutra includes 64 sex positions, where varying difficulties and skill levels are required. Later on, in this book, we will be examining some of these positions in detail, in order for you to get a sense of what positions are included in this sacred text of love. If you enjoy the Kamasutra positions included in this book and want to explore, even more, there are plenty of others for you to try once you master those included in this book.

History of the Kama Sutra

The Kama Sutra is an ancient book that was written in northern India in the language of Ancient Sanskrit. This book was written somewhere between 400 BCE and 200 CE. It was written by an Indian philosopher named Vatsyayana. The word Kama Sutra translates to mean desire, sex, love, or pleasure (*Kama*) book (*Sutra*). More succinctly, Kama sutra means "teachings on desire." This definition of the book title gives great insight into its contents, aside from just the sex positions. Since the book was written so long ago, it was only translated into the English language in 1883. It was then that people in Britain began to learn about The Kama Sutra.

Around the 60's and 70's in North America, with the increasing interest in Indian culture, teachings, and thought practices, the Kama Sutra became of great interest as well. With the age of the hippies and "free love" came the interest in the sex positions contained in the book. People loved the adventurous nature of the sex positions and the variety that they could bring to this new era of sex-positivity. Because of this, the Kama Sutra became known only for the sex positions it contained and not for all of the other chapters on love, romance, and relationships. These other sections include Flirting and courtship, adultery, caste and class, intimacy, and foreplay, as well as same-sex and group-sex.

The Kama Sutra Today

The Kama Sutra is seen today in popular culture as a kinky and fun book to reference in magazine articles and in discussions of sex. It is seen as something for the new-age couple to reference for new positions, including acrobatics and flexibility, which will challenge them and is a great place to start when exploring kinky sex for the first time. Kama Sutra does not technically fall into the category of kink, but it is seen this way in mainstream culture. For many people who have never tried anything out of the ordinary (missionary, cowgirl, etc.) in the bedroom, the positions contained in the Kama Sutra are quite a departure from what they are used to, which is why it is considered kinky.

For a book written so long ago, it is still quite relevant in terms of its discussions on ways to achieve intimacy and how to treat your partner well in a physical sense. You could say that

Kamasutra is a guide to love and enjoying a pleasurable life with yourself and also with another person. It can be seen as a guide to a long-term relationship or a marriage to keep sex interesting and to try new forms of intimacy.

The discussions in the Kama Sutra of same-sex and group-sex relationships are often poorly translated and have been changed in many of the translations to say that it looks down upon these types of relationships, when in fact it simply explores them and mentions them as alternative types of relationships to heterosexual ones, monogamous ones, or both. Because of its mention of these types of romantic or sexual relationships, the book is able to be more relevant today than many other books of its kind. Most ancient sex books, or even more modern ones focus solely on heterosexual relationships. With the growing acceptance of heterosexual relationships and other types of relationships, this book is more relevant today than a lot of others.

Further, the Kama Sutra focuses on sex for pleasure and not for procreation, which is another area where it differs from most ancient sex books. In the time when this was written, sex was mainly talked about as something that happens between two married people in order to continue their bloodline and pass on their status. In this book, however, its talk of pleasure makes it much more relevant to modern relationships and views on sex than many people would think. In a time where people are more sex-positive and adventurous than ever before, the Kama Sutra can align with these views to give relevant sex and relationship guidance even in 2019. Its discussions of sex come from a perspective of sexual freedom for the woman, and for its time, this was very novel, which makes it fitting for today's societies. The Kama Sutra is supportive and encouraging of the female orgasm, which is a new concept even now.

The Benefits of Kama Sutra

There are many benefits of Kama Sutra, some of which are often overlooked. In this section, we will look at the benefits of Kama Sutra including how it can improve not only your sex life but your relationship in general.

Intimacy and Foreplay

The Kama Sutra includes many points for how to love your partner and how to take care of them in non-sexual ways. These ways include how to give good massages of various parts of the body, including the head and the shoulders, the best positions for cuddling that lead to maximum intimacy, and the ways in which you can initiate and carry out foreplay. Because of all of these instructions, you are able to learn more than just show to have an orgasm, and it is focused on more than just the act of sexual intercourse. This is beneficial for a relationship because there are so many resources for sex positions on the internet and in print, but not so many for how to have a tender and loving relationship aside from sex. Reading the sections of the Kama Sutra that are concerned with intimacy and foreplay will benefit your relationship in a number of ways.

Think back on the previous chapter, where we talked about intimacy and the ways that it can benefit your relationship. To achieve greater intimacy, you can learn techniques and methods in the Kama Sutra that will help you get there.

Keeping it Interesting

Another benefit of the Kama Sutra is that it gives you such a multitude of ways to keep your relationship and your sex life interesting. In a long-term relationship, you may feel that you are becoming bored or that your sex life is becoming stale. By reading through the Kama Sutra in its entirety, you can discover ways to keep not only your sex life but your relationship interesting. Maybe you will find a new way to massage or cuddle that you hadn't considered before. Maybe you will find a new technique for oral sex that your partner will love. There are techniques like this for improving your relationship as a whole by keeping it new and interesting.

Chapter 3
How to Prepare the Mind and Body for Sex

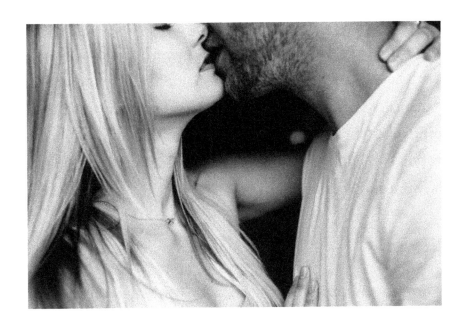

In this chapter, we are going to delve into our study of sex and sex positions by looking at a variety of topics involving the ways in which you can get your mind and body ready for sex. We will look at different parts of sex, including foreplay, as well as orgasm and different ways to pleasure a woman.

The Art of Exciting a Woman: Mind and Body

When it comes to female pleasure, there is a lot to know as many factors are at play. For a woman, her pleasure and her orgasm are very nuanced in what makes them happen. A lot of things can influence the orgasm of a woman, and in this section, we will look at what you can do to optimize a woman's pleasure and her orgasm.

Mind

A woman's mindset plays a big role in whether or not she is able to reach orgasm. If she is distracted or stressed, she may have a difficult time achieving orgasm or even becoming sexually aroused. For this reason, it is important to know how to excite both a woman's mind and her body in order to help her get in the mood for sex.

Setting the Mood

When it comes to setting the mood, women need an environment and an overall ambiance that feels relaxing, sexual, and sensual. To play into your partner's sexual centers in her brain, be sure to set the mood. The reason that this is important is that it will make her feel relaxed and comfortable being vulnerable. She will need to feel comfortable and relaxed in this space in order for her to reach her full arousal potential. Taking some time to set the mood before you have sex will go a long way in terms of her ability to become and stay aroused. As a couple, it is more important to set the mood and environment before having sex than it would be if you were having casual sex or a one-night stand. This is because you are likely together a lot of the time, and in order to transition from regular movie watching to sensual sex time, you will need to change some things.

When setting the mood, your focus is on creating an environment free of distractions where you can both focus on each other without becoming side-tracked. Another focus is to create an environment that is relaxing and calm. This will allow you to get in touch with your sensations and your deeper feelings in order to embrace your pleasure and move in ways that feel good to you, without your thoughts running too much. Sometimes your thoughts can end up running rampant, which will prevent you from being present in the moment and can get in the way of you listening to your body and its needs.

If you are having sex in your bedroom or in your home, it is a space that is very familiar to both of you. This may mean that all of your regular distractions are present all over the place, including your phone, your computer, and your textbooks or your work, maybe. You don't want these things staring at you from across the room, reminding you that you have to study all night or send a quick email after your orgasm is over, so try to keep the room as free of these things as possible. Maybe leave your phone and laptop in the kitchen or the office, and make sure you put it on silent!

Further, because you want the environment to be relaxing, get rid of the harsh lighting of your overhead bulbs and turn on a few lamps with a soft orange glow or light some candles. You don't necessarily have to go so far as having rose petals and chocolates, but some candles will be a nice touch for any day of the week. Setting the mood in this way will allow you both to breathe and focus on each other and yourselves. We all deserve to have some time with our partner and our own bodies, where we just enjoy some pleasure. Use your sex time with your partner as a way to de-stress and let yourself unwind and have some fun. Now that the mood is set, the foreplay can begin.

Easing into the Mindset

It is important that you spend time together getting into the mood. If you rush into sex, it may be difficult for the woman to get her mind into the mood. Spending enough time together to be romantic, to connect, and to relax together will make it so that even before foreplay, the woman is able to relax and focus on herself and on her partner. You can do this in a number of ways. You can do this by spending time talking to each other over a drink, by having a relaxing steamy shower together or by spending time cuddling in bed before taking it up a notch. By doing this even before beginning any foreplay, you will be able to unwind together. This is especially important at the end of a long day.

When it comes to mindset, recognizing that both of you can play an equal part in helping her to reach pleasure and orgasm is beneficial in that you can be aware of things you can do when it proves difficult for her to relax and let go. Both of you can keep in mind that this needs to be done and can begin putting this into practice so that the best sexual experience possible can be had by both of you.

Body

When it comes to the body of a woman, there are many different areas that can be stimulated in many different ways in order to make her feel pleasure. Knowing which areas these are and how to touch them will go a long way in getting a woman aroused and giving her an orgasm.

Firstly, we will look at the different areas of a woman's body from which she can experience sexual pleasure.

Nipples

Every woman is different in how sensitive her nipples are, but many women are able to become very sexually aroused by having their nipples stimulated. This is a good place to start when the moment is just beginning to heat up. It has been reported that some women are even able to reach orgasm through nipple stimulation. If your partner enjoys having her nipples stimulated, she may be one of those!

Labia

The labia are sometimes referred to as the "lips" of a woman's genitals. These structures are located outside of a woman's vagina, and they have some resemblance to lips. There are two sets of labia on a woman's body, the inner and the outer labia. There are two small labia located directly outside of the vaginal opening, which protect the vagina itself from outside debris. There are also the outer labia, which cover the inner labia, the clitoris, and the vagina and protect them all. All of these structures between a woman's legs act to protect the most sensitive and precious areas of her body. While these structures act as protection, they also contain many nerve endings, which make them very sensitive to touch and can, therefore, give the woman immense pleasure when stimulated in the right way. The labia can be stimulated by a man's pelvic region or the base of his penis when he is penetrating her, or when giving her oral sex by using his mouth and facial region. They can also be stimulated by fingers or hands during foreplay or any time the man is using his hands to stimulate the woman's genitals.

Clitoris

The clitoris is the key to pleasure for a woman. The clitoris is sometimes referred to as the female penis. This is because when a woman becomes sexually aroused, her clitoris will fill with blood and swell, causing it to increase in size, much like the penis of a male. When this happens, you can think of like a female erection. What this means is that the enlarging or erection of the clitoris makes it much more sensitive than it normally would be, which leads to feelings of sexual arousal and pleasure when it is touched in the right way. Doing this for some time in the right way can lead to orgasm. In these ways, the clitoris is very similar to the penis of a man.

If you have a female partner or if you are a woman yourself, you have likely had some experience with stimulating the clitoris. Each woman is different in terms of how she likes her clitoris touched and what makes it feel good. This is where communication comes in. You can try different angles, amounts of pressure and speeds to find what makes her moan in pleasure in response. She can also help you to find her clitoris.

When trying to find the clitoris, the following method will prove useful. This can be done by the woman herself if she is trying to find her own clitoris or by the man during the exploration of the woman's body. The woman should lie down on her back whether it is her exploring her own body or having the man do it. The clitoris is located right where the labia or vaginal lips begin, closest to the front side of her body. Begin with your hand pressed to her stomach below her belly button. Pressing two fingers into the skin with gentle pressure, slide your hand down the front of her body, coming closer and closer to the vulva (vulva: general vaginal area). Using your two fingers, feel around as your hand descends, for a small bean-like structure. You may need to move some of her skin around- everyone has different amounts of skin down there so keep feeling around if you do not feel it right away. If your hands reach the vagina and you still have not found the clitoris, begin again at her belly button, and work your way down, this time trying to feel a little deeper in. It may take you a few tries but be patient. Eventually, you will feel the small lump that is the key to the female orgasm. If it proves to be extra difficult, try getting the woman a little bit horny before trying again by watching a sexy video, reading a hot erotica story, or having a hot make-out session. Being aroused will make the clitoris easier to find because, as you know, with sexual arousal, it will become slightly enlarged. When you have found the clitoris, you can then begin to touch it in different ways and find out how exactly it works and what makes it feel good.

Since the clitoris and labia are so closely located to each other and are both very sensitive to erotic touch, they can be stimulated at the same time, and this will give the woman great pleasure when stimulated together.

The Vagina and the G-Spot

The vagina is another sensitive spot on a woman that can give her great feelings of pleasure when physically stimulated. The vagina is a canal located between a woman's legs, which leads to the woman's uterus inside her body. It is, for this reason, that sex can lead to pregnancy because at the end of the vagina are all of her reproductive parts. (Not to worry though, if you are using proper protection you shouldn't have to worry about that). The walls of the vagina contain several places that, when stimulated, will lead to very intense orgasms for the woman. You have likely heard of the G-Spot before. The G-Spot is one of the spots within the vagina that can give a woman an orgasm. This spot can be stimulated with the man's penis during penetration or with fingers.

Since there are different zones within the vagina that can lead to very intense orgasms, we are going to look at how to find one of them. We are going to look at how to find the G-Spot since this is the spot located closest to the vaginal opening and is the easiest to find and the easiest to stimulate with the penis during penetration. The best way to find the G-spot is with the fingers. To find this spot, the man can try finding it which will not only show him where to aim during penetration but will also make the woman feel good while he is exploring. Using fingers will allow him to feel his way more easily around and will give him more control over his movements. To begin, slide your fingers inside of the vagina and tilt your fingers towards the front of the woman's body. Move your fingers up towards the front of her body so that your fingers are making a "come here" motion. You will feel a slightly raised, bumpy surface. Gently pressing on this spot with your fingers should make her feel great. If you are the man that is doing this, communicate with her to see if you have found the spot.

It does not have to be the man doing this exploration if the woman would rather be the one to find the G-Spot. The woman can find it inside of herself either when masturbating or when with a partner. The woman can feel for this small, bumpy surface on the inside of her own vagina on the front-most wall of the body. This spot is the G-Spot. If either of you are having difficulty finding this spot, similar to the clitoris, the G-spot becomes raised when the woman is sexually aroused, and this will help you to find it and to stimulate it. Only a small part of the clitoris can be seen from the outside of the body, but the majority of this structure extends into the inside of the body, like the tip of an iceberg. As it happens, the part of the clitoris that extends inside of the woman's body can be felt inside of the vagina. This part of the clitoris inside of the vagina is actually the G-Spot. As I mentioned, when a woman is aroused, her clitoris enlarges. Therefore, her G-Spot also enlarges, and this makes it easier to find and easier to stimulate when she is aroused. If you are trying to find the G-Spot and trying to give a woman a G-Spot orgasm, doing so when she is aroused will be the best time to do so.

There are certain positions that make for the optimal angles of penis-to-vagina for G-Spot stimulation, and we will look at these later on in this book. For now, it is important to note that when stimulated the G-Spot will lead to a very intense and extremely pleasurable orgasm for the woman. In order for this to happen, though, the exact spot must be stimulated repeatedly as her pleasure builds all the way until it reaches a climax, and she orgasms. This is why, at first, it is best to use fingers until you both understand just how to make the most of the G-Spot.

The Anus

The anus is a less well-known and less discussed spot that contains many pleasure centers for a woman. A woman is able to become very sexually aroused and feel great sexual pleasure from having her anus stimulated. An anal orgasm is not something that the majority of women have experience with, but it is one that can be very pleasurable for her. This type of orgasm takes some time to occur, as the anus is a very sensitive part of the body, but when done in the right way, a woman can experience a full-blown orgasm. This stimulation leading to orgasm can include either or both the outside of the anus and just inside the anal canal. This can happen using a penis, fingers, a toy, or a person's mouth.

You may already be aware that when it comes to anal sex or anal play of any sort, there are some things to keep in mind to maximize pleasure and minimize pain or discomfort of any sort. Firstly, anal sex requires a lot of lube since the anus cannot lubricate itself in the way that the vagina can. Ensuring you have enough lubrication is important in minimizing discomfort and maximizing pleasure. Secondly, when having anal sex, especially for the first time, you will need to take it slowly. There is no need to rush. The key is to ensure the woman is comfortable with the depth and speed of penetration before going deeper or faster. The anus will relax and widen as you stimulate it more, so be patient. This is important no matter what you are using to penetrate her anally. Begin by stimulating the outer rim of her anus using your mouth or your fingers (with lube), and then as the anus relaxes, you can begin to penetrate slowly and gently. When she is comfortable with all of this and is feeling pleasure, you can begin to slowly penetrate her anally. If she is feeling any pain or discomfort at any point, stop what you are doing and adjust so that she is comfortable. The goal is pleasure!

Foreplay

Foreplay is always seen as the preamble to sex. It has a reputation of being the part of sex that you want to speed through in order to get to the "good stuff." But when you think about it, do any of us really want to just stick it in and be done with sex only minutes later? Sex between couples is much more than a *pump and dump,* and some of the best parts of sex when in a relationship can happen during foreplay. Treating sex as an emotionally intimate act and not just a physical one means that we need to treat all parts of it-including foreplay, with just as much importance as the actual act of penis-in-vagina sex. Foreplay gives you the chance to connect emotionally before you begin connecting physically in such a deep way. This can be the difference between lovemaking and just the physical act of sex. In this section, we will look at foreplay as a special part of sex and the reasons why it is such a necessary part of sex for both people involved.

Foreplay's Importance for the Female Orgasm

Foreplay is extremely important and necessary for a woman to reach orgasm. While women can become aroused by visual stimuli, it is hard for them to reach a point where their body is ready for penetration and orgasm from this alone. Women require extra time leading up to the point of penetration by a penis. This is so that penetration is more enjoyable for her, as this gives her time to get adequately wet so that the man's penis is able to slide in and out of her smoothly.

During foreplay is when you caress, grope, make out with and touch each other. This is when the woman will become very aroused from the man's touch. Giving her time to feel pleasure from physical touch and to let these sensations build will allow her to become aroused enough to reach orgasm at some point during sex. If it is too rushed, she will not have enough time to let her pleasure take over her body, and she will likely have a difficult time getting all the way there.

By taking your time and touching the woman in a variety of ways, getting her more and more aroused, you may be able to bring her to orgasm during foreplay. While this is great for the woman, it is also great for foreplay in general as this will, without a doubt, lead her to become extremely wet. This wetness will mean that her vagina and her mind are ready for penetrative sex. The more aroused a woman becomes, the greater the potential of a G-spot orgasm during penetration. As you now know, when a woman becomes aroused, her erogenous zones swell with pleasure, and this makes it easier for them to be physically stimulated by the penis or by fingers. Giving the woman an orgasm during foreplay will increase her level of arousal by a large amount, which will make penetrative sex that much better for both of you. When a woman is very aroused, and her vagina swells with blood, this tightens the canal, and the man can feel this effect on his penis. This is why the more aroused the woman, the better the sex for both of them.

The Orgasm

We have discussed the female orgasm somewhat in this chapter so far, but in this section, we will look at it in a little more depth.

For a woman to reach orgasm, much of this is dependent on her mindset. She will need to feel comfortable being vulnerable in this space in order for her to reach her full arousal potential. She needs to reach this point in order for her to orgasm and in order for her to fully enjoy sex. For this reason, mindset and pleasure are very closely linked to a woman.

The Clitoral Orgasm

When the clitoris is rubbed in the right way, it will lead to orgasm, just like the penis of a man. Treating it like this can give both men and women insight into how it works and how to make the woman come. When stimulated physically with someone's fingers or a sex toy like a vibrator, this can lead to an orgasm for the woman. The clitoris is a structure that contains many nerve endings, which is what makes it so sensitive. When a woman is not aroused sexually, her clitoris is still there, but it will not be as enlarged as when she is horny.

Vaginal Pleasure

As we discussed in the section regarding foreplay, a woman's vagina automatically swells when she is sexually aroused because of increased blood flow to her genitals, sort of like how your penis becomes erect when you get horny. What this means for you is that when your penis is inside of her, the walls of her vagina will tighten and swell as the blood flow increases, and you will feel this effect on your penis, resulting in added pleasure for you.

Multiple Orgasms

There are different types of multiple orgasms that a woman can achieve. Women are lucky in that they are able to have both back-to-back orgasms and blended orgasms. They are even able to have back-to-back blended orgasms in some cases! In this section, we will learn more about the different types of multiple orgasms.

Blended Orgasms

We will now discuss blended orgasms. A blended orgasm is achieved when multiple different orgasms are achieved at the same time. This can be two different orgasms at the same time, or in some cases, even more than two! This type of orgasm leads to even more pleasure than a single orgasm and will lead the woman to feel more intense pleasure than ever before. During penetration, there is lots of opportunity for different types of female orgasms to occur. The two most common ways that a woman can reach orgasm are through her clitoris and through her G-spot. We will look at some ways that a woman can have both of these orgasms at the same time, as well as some other options for blended orgasms.

Any combination of these separate but simultaneous orgasms compound to give the woman a mind-blowing, full-body, blended orgasm. This is especially so if the two locations of stimulation are a larger distance from each other- like the nipples and the clitoris, for example. The best type of blended orgasm will vary from woman to woman, depending on her personal preferences and what her most sensitive erogenous zones are. Some of these zones include the clitoris, the anus, the G-Spot, and the nipples. Some women may have others as well, but this is largely dependent on the woman's body.

Clitoral and G-Spot Blended Orgasm

The first method is a clitoral orgasm during penetration. If the clitoris is stimulated while the man is penetrating the woman, it is possible that she can have an orgasm through both her clitoris and her G-Spot at the same time. This type of multiple orgasm will make her feel pleasure like never before because these two places are extremely pleasurable even when achieved alone, so together, it is a new level of orgasm! There are different ways that you can achieve this, but the most successful way is to penetrate her with your fingers while she rubs her clitoris at the same time. This way, you can feel your way around and stimulate her G-spot while she pleases herself. It may take some practice and will require a lot of communication, but eventually, you will both be able to time it so that she can have both of these orgasms at once. Another way that this can happen is while the man is thrusting his penis into her. While he is doing this, she can touch her clitoris using her fingers or a vibrator, or the man can stimulate her clitoris by using his fingers or a vibrator. There are also some specific positions that will allow for the man's penis to reach the G-Spot when inside of her, and at the same time, the base of his penis or his pelvic region can rub her clitoris, causing both orgasms to happen at the same time. We will look at these specific positions later on in this book.

Anal and Clitoral Blended Orgasm

Another way that a woman can achieve a blended orgasm is through having both an anal and a clitoral orgasm at the same time. This is similar to the blended orgasm in which the man is penetrating the woman with his penis while her clitoris is being stimulated, but in this case, it is done while you are having anal sex. The method will happen in a similar way to the vaginal penetration with clitoral stimulation, but the positions used will be slightly different as the positions used in this case would be ones that better allow for anal penetration while giving either the man or the woman free hands to stimulate the clitoris. Either the man or the woman can stimulate the woman's clitoris in a variety of anal sex positions using either their hands or a vibrating sex toy.

Nipple and Clitoral Blended Orgasm

Another type of blended orgasm that is possible is a nipple orgasm and a clitoral orgasm. Not every woman is able to achieve a nipple orgasm, but if you are, then this could be a great option for a blended orgasm. If you are unsure whether you are able to reach orgasm through nipple stimulation alone, try this one in order to see if also having your clitoris stimulated leads to more sensitivity in your nipples as well.

One example of a position in which this type of blended orgasm can occur is the following. While you are sitting in a chair with your legs spread wide, your partner will get on his knees in front of you. He will then begin to give you oral sex on his knees. While licking and using his mouth to stimulate your clitoris, he will reach up to your breasts with his hands and massage your nipples with his fingers. Once he has done this for some time and began to please you, he will then switch and using his tongue. He will gently lick, suck, and flick your nipples with his tongue, one at a time. While he does this, he will also move his hand down between your legs and stimulate your clitoris with his hand and fingers. Have him alternate back and forth using his mouth on your clitoris and then on your nipples. This will give you pleasure from both of these erogenous zones, and you will likely be able to experience a blended nipple and clitoral orgasm in this way, as long as he keeps stimulating both areas at the same time.

Back-to-Back Orgasms

Not only can women have blended orgasms, but they can also have back-to-back orgasms. These orgasms occur one after the other and give the woman immense pleasure because she is able to keep coming again and again and again.

This type of repeated orgasm is only possible for women as the male body is unable to do this. This is due to the fact that the male body has to wait for a refractory period after every orgasm. What this means is that there is an amount of time after an orgasm during which a man's body is unable to achieve an erection or have another orgasm. During this time, his body is recovering from the orgasm and needs this time to recuperate. The length of this period is different for every man, but it ranges between fifteen to thirty minutes in most males.

The great thing about the clitoris is that after orgasm, it may be very sensitive for a few minutes, but it maintains its "erection" and can be stimulated again a very short time after for a doubly-pleasurable second orgasm. This can lead to a third and a fourth and beyond. This is why, as we discussed, it is beneficial to give a woman an orgasm during foreplay as it will increase her chances of orgasm during penetration because of how horny it will have made her. Sometimes, women's pleasure only builds after an initial orgasm instead of going back to zero before climbing again like a man's pleasure would have to. It is important for men to understand this difference because they can then take advantage of it and pleasure their woman to the fullest. While they await their refractory period, they can please their woman in a way that does not involve their penis, give her an orgasm, and then by the time this happens. He will be ready to get hard again and have a second round with her. All the while, she will become increasingly horny and pleased.

Simultaneous Orgasms

Another type of multiple orgasm that may be different from what you had in mind when hearing the words "multiple orgasms" is the simultaneous orgasm." This type of multiple orgasm is great for couples, especially long-term couples. This type of orgasm occurs when both the man and the woman are able to reach orgasm at the same time! The reason why this is great for long-term couples is that it takes practice and excellent communication during sex, but when mastered, it will unlock new levels of pleasure for both of you. When in a long-term relationship, one of the many positive things about having sex with each other is that you know just the right way to make each other orgasm. After having sex with each other so many times, you likely have this down to a science! This comes in handy here as you can use this knowledge to help you both orgasm at the same time. Since you know how to get your partner to orgasm in mere minutes, you can touch each other exactly as you each like at the exact same time in order to reach orgasm simultaneously.

Now, this is a little more difficult than it sounds, but it is entirely possible. To do this, begin with the intention of orgasming together. Both of you will stimulate the other person's genitals in the best way you know, so you will have to figure out a position that allows for both of these ways at the same time. For example, if your partner can make you come very quickly by giving you oral sex while also massaging your testicles and you can make her come very quickly by playing with her clitoris just the right way, then you will have to find a position where you can do both of these at the same time. This position could be one where you are lying on your back on the bed, and she is straddling your chest, facing your feet. She will bend forward so that her mouth reaches your penis, and she will hold herself up with one of her arms on the bed. She can then use her other free hand to massage your testicles. You will then slide a hand between her legs and begin playing with her clitoris, and you can even use your other hand to slide your fingers into her vagina if she wishes.

When you begin, start out slow. This will require a lot of communication between the two of you. Begin pleasing each other and communicating your pleasure with moans or simple phrases like "that feels good" the entire time. When one of you gets close to reaching orgasm, tell the other person. If your partner tells you that they are close to coming, ease up on the pressure or the speed on her clitoris, for example, so that she does not come yet. When, and if you are also close to orgasm, let her know, and you can both continue to stimulate each other's genitals until you both orgasms together at the same time!

One of the benefits of this type of orgasm in a long-term relationship is that when you care about a person deeply, you find pleasure in seeing them pleased. When you please your partner to the point of orgasm, it usually will make you also feel pleasure. Because of this, as each of you comes closer to reaching orgasm, it will make the other person more aroused. For this reason, a long-term couple will be able to do this act of simultaneous orgasms with ease.

Female Ejaculation

Female ejaculation is a well-disputed concept in modern discussions about sexuality. There is evidence, though, that it is possible and actually quite common. While the term *female ejaculation* probably makes you think of something porn-related, it is something that can happen without theatrics and to a much lesser degree in your own sex life. Female ejaculation is often portrayed as a fountain of water spraying across the room; however, this is not the case in real life.

Female ejaculation does not have to occur, and, in many cases, it never does. It is sort of the icing on the cake or the cherry on top, so to speak, but it is not necessary in order for the woman to be aroused or to achieve orgasm. Female ejaculation, commonly referred to as *squirting,* is different for every woman and does not have to involve a large amount of fluid like a male ejaculation. It also does not happen every time and does not only happen during orgasm. While it can happen at the time of orgasm, female ejaculation can also occur at any time during sex when the woman is extremely aroused. Thus, ejaculation can be a sign that the woman is feeling aroused regardless of whether she has reached orgasm yet or not. This is a good sign that indicates she is enjoying herself.

Ejaculation does not happen to every woman, but it can be something that can be practiced and learned if the woman would like to experience it. Some people become extremely turned on when they experience or witness female ejaculation, so if you or your partner feel that it would turn you both on, it is possible for the woman to begin trying to achieve this. For some people, it turns them on so much, even to the point of experiencing orgasm.

Female ejaculation has been linked to G-Spot stimulation, so the best way to achieve this is to have your partner stimulate your G-Spot with either his fingers, his penis, or a dildo.

Chapter 4
Unlocking Your Sexual Fantasies and Fetishes

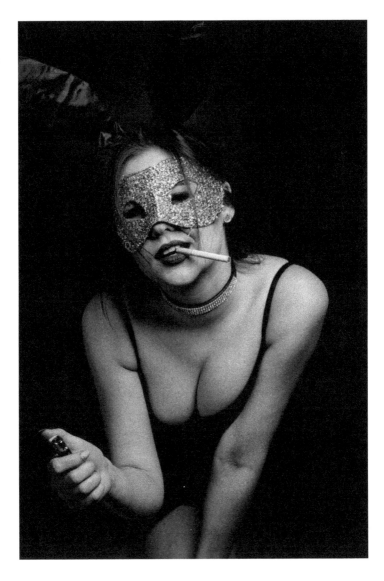

In this chapter, we will look at sexual fantasies, kinks, and fetishes. We will examine them in terms of what they are, how they can come into play in your relationship and how this can ultimately improve your intimacy levels and your sex life. First, we will begin by looking at exactly what these are.

What is a Sexual Fantasy?

A sexual fantasy is something that a person imagines or dreams of doing or taking part in. This fantasy is of a sexual nature as it usually will involve something that you would not regularly have the chance to do. For example, it could be something like having sex with a teacher as their student. In this case, this is not something that you would likely do, but you fantasize about doing it as it arouses you.

What Is a Fetish and What Is a Kink?

The lines between Kink and Fetish can blur, as the level and degree to which you enjoy something sexually can vary greatly. The things that turn people on are different for every individual and every couple, and so the definitions of kink and fetish must be somewhat flexible as well.

A kink is something that arouses you that is not considered to be the norm in your sexual culture. What is considered a kink can vary from culture to culture and between different eras in time? The terms *kink* and *BDSM* can be used somewhat interchangeably these days. Kink generally includes some type of power dynamic and dominance versus submission element. Kink is the opposite of vanilla or basic sex.

Fetishes are different than kinks in that the fetish will be more prominent to you in your arousal and pleasure. The fetish will often be more important than the person that is helping you to carry out your fetish. What this means is that a sexual fetish is a sexual attraction to an object or a body part that would not normally be associated with sexual pleasure, and this becomes a bigger focus in many cases than the partner themselves do. A fetish is required to be played out in one's sexual encounters in order for them to get off and even become aroused in some cases.

Oftentimes, you will see the terms kink and fetish used interchangeably, and this is because it all depends to what degree a person enjoys something.

How to Discover Your Sexual Fantasies and Fetishes

You are now aware of what sexual fantasies and fetishes are, but you may now be wondering if you have any personally.

Everyone has sexual acts or themes that turn them on, but you must get in touch with this part of yourself in order to find out what your personal ones are. In this section, we are going to look at how you can discover your sexual fantasies and fetishes.

First, though, we will look at some specific types of sexual fantasies so that you can get an idea of what you are looking to discover. Under the umbrella of sexual fantasies is included the following, among others;

- ### *Roleplay*

If your sexual fantasy or kink is role play, you likely become aroused when you imagine playing a certain role in the bedroom with your partner like a homeowner, and he is a plumber coming to fix your pipes.

- ### *Domination and Submission*

If your kink or fetish is domination and submission, you likely become turned on by playing a certain role in bed- either being dominated by your partner or being dominant over them.

- ### *Specific Sexual Acts*

Your kink could also be related to specific sexual acts. These can include spanking, hair pulling or Piss Play

There are so many things that can be included in these categories and so many more categories of their own. Many categories will overlap and cross over each other. For example, a police and convict role play fantasy could cross over into domination and submission play as well. By getting an idea of what is out there, you can begin to explore what you like the idea of and what you don't like sexually.

Look Inward

The first part of determining anything about yourself is to look inward and get in touch with your inner thoughts, feelings, and desires. If you are not used to looking inward and examining your feelings, it may take some practice and getting used to before you are able to determine what your fantasies, kinks or fetishes are. In order to get in touch with your feelings and thoughts, set aside some time to get quiet with your own mind.

Start to begin letting yourself fantasize about sex in general and see where this takes you. The main thing here is to let your mind go wherever it goes without trying to control it. By allowing it to drift anywhere and everywhere, you can begin to see what lies hidden in your subconscious mind.

Avoid Self-Judgement

Self-judgement can sometimes creep in when you become sexually aroused by something that is deemed unacceptable in society. When you have a sexual fantasy, it is important to remember that there need not be any shame involved- having a specific sexual fantasy does not mean that you would actually act it out in real life. Because of this, you can put your self-judgments aside and enjoy your fantasy without thinking of yourself as some sort of deviant.

Masturbation

As you are giving yourself a quiet moment to explore your mind and your desires, you may find yourself becoming sexually aroused. This is great, as it means that you have found some things that are sexually exciting to you. As this happens, you can begin to touch yourself if you wish. Masturbation is a healthy part of anybody's sex life, and there is no shame in this either.

As you begin touching yourself, allow your mind to explore your sexual fantasies, kinks, and fetishes more deeply as you become aroused. By doing this, you will be much more able to let your subconscious take over you. This is where your desires and your deeper wishes are held. Most of the time, these remain in your subconscious unbeknownst to you. It is only when you are able to access this part of your mind that you can become aware of what lies there. By doing this, you allow yourself to unlock a different level of sexual adventure and exploration. This is something that you can then share with your partner, and they can begin to know you on a much deeper level.

Research

As I stated earlier, you may not even know what sexual fantasies and fetishes are out there. By doing a little bit of research, you can figure out what is out there, what is encompassed by these terms, and what you specifically find pleasure in.

You can do research in different ways. You could explore different articles on the internet of *The Most Common Sexual Fantasies* or *Stories of the Weirdest Sexual Fetishes*. You could also look at different types of porn as there is an unlimited amount of porn available on the internet, and within this, there is a wide array of fantasies and fetishes included. The one thing to keep in mind when looking at porn is that you want to make sure you are not taking the sex you see in porn as reality. While the ideas of fantasies and fetishes can be informative to you, porn can also set unrealistic expectations for viewers related to things such as average penis size or breast size as well as how to please a woman. As long as you keep this in mind, porn can be a useful tool for exploring kinks and fetishes you never knew existed.

Even if you only find out what you are not interested in sexually, this research will still have proven to be informative.

Talk to People

Talking to your friends or people who you meet that are open about their sex lives can be another great source of information for you. The benefit to this as well is that it can give you a more realistic view of these things than you may be able to find on the internet.

You could begin by asking people about their sexual fantasies, or if they are aware of them at all. You can ask them also if they have shared these with their partners. By initiating a conversation like this, you can learn a lot about other people and their sexual fantasies or kinks.

Once you have begun to explore your sexual fantasies, kinks, and fetishes, you will be able to begin exploring them. There are many ways to try new things in the bedroom for the first time, and we will discuss this in a later section of this chapter. Exploring your fetishes is a lifelong process, as your likes and desires may change over time. Once you have found out how to be in touch with this part of yourself, you can continue to let it inform your sex life forever.

How to Discuss Your Fetishes with Your Partner

It may seem quite intimidating opening up to your partner about your kinks or fetishes or even your sexual fantasies as they are very personal to you. You may fear judgment or disgust, and you may fear that your partner will not be interested in taking part in your sexual fantasies or fetishes. In this section, I will guide you through how you can discuss these things with your partner in an open and honest way without shame or fear.

You may be self-conscious about what turns you on and unsure of how your partner will feel about it. If you have been in this relationship for a while now and you still have not discussed these with your partner, your anxiety about bringing them up has likely only increased with time. At the beginning of a relationship, you may be hesitant to bring up things that please you that you deem unusual or not-so-vanilla. This is completely understandable, and we will discuss how to bring these topics up in conversation, regardless of how long you have been in your current relationship or marriage. The other reason could be that you have just recently discovered a new kink, and that is okay as well. If you have never acted on them before, talking to your partner about trying them can be done as a conversation about mutual exploration.

Keep in mind that many of us think our kinks are odd and embarrassing, but they are probably not as off the wall as you think they are. Fetishes may also be embarrassing to discuss, but if you are so into a certain thing that you require it in order to be pleased, your partner will surely be interested. As your partner, they are invested in your pleasure and should always be wondering how best to please you. So how do you initiate a conversation about your kinks or fetishes with your partner or spouse? The key is entering the conversation with the intention of not only explaining to them your own desires but of listening to and understanding your partner's kinks and fetishes as well.

Begin by asking your partner if there is anything that they have been interested in trying in the bedroom, or if there is anything new that they have wanted to explore sexually with you. This will initiate an open dialogue about sex and desires in general. Listen with an open mind. Your partner may be into something that you are also into! Next, they will likely ask you the same question back. Explain to them that you have wanted to try something new in your sex life with them.

Explain to them what it is and how it makes you feel. Maybe you have explored this in a past relationship, and maybe that is where you first discovered this specific thing that turns you on. Maybe you have never tried it with someone else, and you would like to begin exploring it with them. If this person loves you, they care about your pleasure. Even if they may have reservations about trying something new, they are likely to be open to giving it a shot for you. Be open to exploring your kink or fetish at a beginner level if your partner has never tried it before. Sex is all about comfort and pleasure and as long as you are both feeling these two things, preferably by meeting in the middle, a good time is sure to be had by all. When explaining your kink to them, be sure to explain how it makes you feel and how it could make them feel. Explain what exactly you enjoy about it. Explain how exactly you enjoy it and what role you like to take in it. Do you like to be the dominant one? The submissive one? Allow them to ask questions and be curious. the ability to have an open conversation about sex in a relationship is essential to having a positively evolving sex life as your relationship grows and progresses. You want your sex life to grow and change along with the both of you.

We will now look at an example of this and how this conversation may go for you, in order for you to feel more secure when bringing this up. For example, say your kink is rough sex. You and your partner may have been having soft, gentle, and loving sex up until this point because you know that that is what they like, but you have learned through a past relationship that you love rough sex. You may not have tried this or brought it up in conversation before because you were afraid that your partner would have been turned off or afraid. In order to bring this up to them in conversation, you can begin by saying something like, "I used to get very turned on by having rough sex, and I would like to try it with you."

How to Try New Fantasies and Fetishes for the First Time

When talking to your partner about your fetishes, they will likely be open-minded and willing to try it with you. This is great! In order to do this for the first time, there will be some things to keep in mind.

New Fantasy, Kink, or Fetish for Both People

If you have just discovered a new fetish or a new kink that you wish to try and you have discussed this with your partner, you can now begin to introduce this into your sex life. The positive thing about neither of you have done it before is that it can be an experience that you share with one another. By doing this, you can both evaluate as you go and decide what you like and what you dislike. For example, if you are wishing to try out a role play, you can begin by getting into the roles and using dirty talk as your characters, while ensuring that you have a safe word to use just in case someone becomes uncomfortable. A safeword is a predetermined word that you or your partner can say when one of you wishes to put the play aside and become yourselves for a time. You can use this to tell your partner that you wish to stop, to change something or to tell them something out of character. This can be used for any kink, fetish, or fantasy that you are playing out.

New Fantasy, Kink, or Fetish for Your Partner Only

If you have experience with the kink, fetish, or fantasy, but your partner does not, we will look at how to try this with your partner for the first time here.

Continuing with the example in the previous section, if you are bringing up your fetish with your partner and this fetish is rough sex, there are many ways that you can begin to introduce this into your sex life with your partner without going straight to BDSM, as they may be a little afraid in the beginning and wish to ease into it, though they are open-minded. This is completely okay. There are many degrees of roughness in sex, and it will be easy to start out by just dipping your toes in the world of rough sex to see how your partner feels about it. You can explain this to them as well. Once they are comfortable with the idea and are wanting to try it with you, you will need to take the lead. Your partner will probably not know where to start, and you will lead them through it for their first few times. To teach them as you go, try using dirty talk to make it sexier than if you just gave them a lesson in kink like a lecture at school. Begin by explaining to them whether you enjoy being in the position of masochist (pleasure from pain inflicted on you) or sadist (pleasure from inflicting pain on another person). For example, you may like having your hair pulled or having your partner dig their nails into your back when you make them feel good.

Begin by having sex as you usually would, and when it comes time that you would like it to get a little rougher, tell your partner(using dirty talk) what you want them to do. Say something like the following; "pull my hair baby" or "spank me like you're punishing me". This will make your directions sexy and fitting for the mood. Your partner may be afraid to hurt you if they do not have experience with rough sex. You can assure them before you begin that they will not be hurting you, but in fact, they will be making you feel more pleasure than usual. They will likely be excited by this possibility. This may be enough for the first time, but be sure to communicate in order to find this out. Every person is different so every person's comfort level will be different. Your partner may get into it and end up loving it just as much as you do. By beginning in this way, you can go a little further each time you have sex, and in this way, both people's comfort and enjoyment are considered.

Chapter 5
Tantric Sex

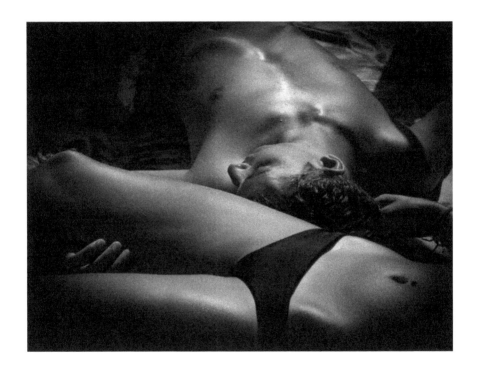

I this chapter, we are going to move on to another type of sex called Tantric sex. If you have never heard of this type of sex before, we are going to start with a little introduction.

What Is Tantric Sex?

Tantric sex is derived from something called the Tantra, which is a very old spiritual practice. For our purposes, we will be primarily looking at how the Tantra practice relates to sex and not at the other facets of this type of spirituality, though they are inextricably linked. In the way that Tantra has become related to sex, it can be viewed as a sort of new-age or *Neo-Tantra*. This is a modern take on Tantra that links it to sex and sex positions that we hear about most often today in the Western World.

Tantric Sex or Neotantra is essentially spiritual sex. It takes the old beliefs and teachings of Tantra and brings them into our modern relationships, and sex lives in order to help us better connect in our romantic relationships and to be one with our bodies and sensations. This type of sex is great for couples and long-term relationships. One of the main focuses of Tantric Sex is a mutual exchange of energy between partners. Another focus is getting in touch with the sensations and feelings of your body. It is also about removing distractions and being mindful in order to have more intense, longer-lasting, full-body orgasms. Being mindful means to bring your consciousness and awareness to the present moment. It is the state of being fully present in your body, your actions, and thoughts, and noticing them as they change. Being in this state allows you to feel the physical sensations within your body and removes the distraction of a mind full of running thoughts.

The Science Behind Tantric Sex

In Tantric Sex, everything comes down to the belief that women are generally taught to always focus on the needs of others and on taking care of others, as well as to place more importance on the pleasure of others than on themselves. It is believed that women are so disconnected from their feelings and sensations that they must begin a practice of mindfulness in order to reconnect with their feelings and sensations.

Tantric Theory states that women have a more difficult time than men when it comes to reaching orgasm. Specifically, it states that women are quite preoccupied with the duties of the household, including the children and their needs, the household and its needs, their work, their friends, and anything and anyone else in their lives. They are also preoccupied with subtle distractions such as noises or the temperature, demonstrating that they are always on high alert in an attempt to ensure everything is running smoothly and that nobody is uncomfortable in any way. This is similar to what we discussed when we looked at how to get in the right mindset for sex in terms of removing distractions and prioritizing foreplay.

In short, Tantric theory is of the belief that women are raised to focus on the pleasure and wellbeing of others and are as a result, out of touch completely with their own bodies, their own pleasure, and their own desires (these desires can be both of a sexual nature and otherwise, but here, we will focus on the sexual desires). Because of this, when it comes to sex, women tend to be unable to put aside their focus on others and turn that focus inward to themselves. When in a long-term relationship, they will be so invested in the pleasure of their partner that they will not focus on their own. Even in a casual sexual encounter, the woman will be focused on ensuring that she is giving the man a good time at the expense of her own pleasure.

To further its theories on the attention of women and their focus on many outside factors during sex, Tantric theory states that even if she wanted to, she would not have the ability to turn her focus inward. The belief is that women are unable to get in touch with the sensations of their body or their sexual desires because they have been raised to always put those aside, thus never developing the skills to do so. If she is not able to get in touch with these parts of herself, she will have great difficulty reaching orgasm. This is because she will have difficulty actually feeling what she is feeling, what she likes and doesn't like, and what she wants her partner to do in order to give her an orgasm. She will likely even have difficulty reaching orgasm when she is alone for the same reasons.

Tantric theory also has a theory concerning men and their pleasure. It is believed that men generally have short and intense orgasms and that it is possible for them to have better and longer-lasting orgasms through the practice of mindfulness as well. Tantra focuses on teaching men to be able to prolong their orgasms and make them more all-encompassing as well as to extend their pleasure overall.

Tantric sex has many techniques and methods for overcoming these challenges, and its main intention concerning women is to help them refocus their attention to themselves and their body's sensations. By refocusing on their bodies, it allows women to fully access the parts of their brain related to sexual arousal without just as equally activating the parts of their brain related to worry and concern for others.

The practice of Tantra, in general, involves being in touch with one's feelings and one's breath- almost like a meditation. Neotantra or Tantric Sex takes this idea and uses it in relation to sex. Sex with oneself or sex with a partner is done through a deep connection to oneself and one's partner. In order to do this, you practice being connected to yourself and your deeper feelings in order to feel all of the sensations in your body more easily and reach orgasm quicker and with more intensity.

Tantric sex is so useful for couples, especially those who have been together for some time. At the beginning of your relationship, you were connected by the lust, the exploration of each other, and the excitement. Now, since you know each other so well, it can be hard to reach that same feeling of discovery in the bedroom. Tantric sex can help you get there.

For men, Tantric Sex aims to help them to fully feel and enjoy their orgasms, to make them more intense and longer-lasting and to make them build up much more before releasing. It teaches women to be more present in their pleasure and as a result, their orgasms. Accomplishing these things as well as reaching a greater level of intimacy with your partner is sure to bring you to a new level of connection within your relationship, no matter how long you have been together. Devote yourselves to this practice over time (it won't happen overnight), and it will give you something to work towards as a couple and get you excited about sex with each other again.

Tantric Massage Techniques

Tantric massage is a very common way to practice tantric sex. This massage can be on one of the genital areas such as the testicles, the penis, the vulva, the nipples, and so on, or it can be done on the head or shoulders. The intention here regardless of where the massage takes place, is to focus on your breathing and get into a state of mindfulness. When you can do this, you will feel each of your partner's fingers putting gentle pressure into your skin and the sensations that this produces inside of you. By being in this state during the massage, it is a great way to get your body ready to experience sex in a deeper way, which will greatly increase the chances and intensity of orgasm.

Yoni Massage

A Yoni Massage is a vaginal massage that is intended to open up the woman to her sexuality, her pleasure, and her sexual desires. As a partner, you can perform this type of massage for your woman to unlock her repressed sexual energy and help her to get in touch with it.

This can be done in a variety of ways, but the position we are going to discuss is a Hot Water Yoni Massage. Begin by setting the ambiance, either in the bathroom with a bathtub, or around your jacuzzi. Set up some candles, some flowers, or anything that will make the surroundings relaxing and calm. Begin by having her breathe deeply and focus on her body and its sensations. You can get into the water with her for added intimacy. Begin by slowly and gently massaging around her entire vulva and her clitoral area. The key to this type of massage is to do everything very slowly. Begin to massage her clitoris slowly and not with the intention of making her come. When ready, and with lots of waterproof lube, slide one finger inside of her vagina and gently begin massaging the upper wall. Here is where her G-spot is located. Encourage her to express and release any sounds she naturally makes. Move your finger in a circular motion slowly and with your other hand, massage her pelvic area and clitoris. This connects the inner with the outer. Continue to do this and let the experience unfold with no end goal in mind. If she reaches orgasm, she can do so, but if she doesn't, she can just enjoy the pleasures that she is getting from your massage. As discussed earlier, this massage is intended to reconnect a woman with her pleasure and allow her to focus on herself and her body. After this massage, she will feel more in touch with her body, and if penetrative sex ensues, both of you will feel even more pleasure and intensity of orgasms because of how engorged and activated her vagina and clitoris will be. After doing this practice for some time either with you or on her own, she will be more in tune with her body all of the time and not just when doing this practice. This will lead to stronger orgasms overall and hotter sex for both of you.

Whatever direction this takes afterward (sex or no sex), being able to connect with your partner in this physical and energetic way will be beneficial to your sex life and your relationship as a whole. It can help the woman to reach orgasm during penetration because both of your bodies will have formed a deep connection where the pleasure is able to build both independently and together. Both of you will be in touch with your own and each other's bodies, while also being comfortable allowing your body to feel whatever it may feel and being present enough in the moment to welcome this.

Tantra is an ancient practice that has been helping couples to reconnect for decades. While you may not see yourself as someone who practices specific meditation or spiritual techniques of any sort, or if you tend to relate to more modern ideas, you may be wondering if Tantra is for you. The way that Tantra has been incorporated into sex and sexuality is actually quite a modern approach to Tantra, but nevertheless, there is a reason that its beliefs and techniques remain virtually unchanged after all this time.

Chapter 6

Aphrodisiacs

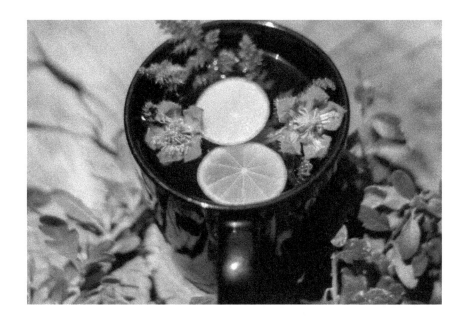

In this chapter, we are going to talk about something that can spice up your relationship and bring a new element of fun and excitement to your sex life as a couple. This new element is called an Aphrodisiac! Below, I will explain what they are and how you can incorporate them into your sex life.

What are They?

An aphrodisiac is a food or a substance that, when ingested, leads people to become sexually aroused. Many people will use these as a fun and flirty way to get them and or their partner in the mood for sex.

Aphrodisiacs work by affecting specific parts of the body, depending on which food or substance you ingest, which causes sexual arousal as a result. They can work in one of the following two ways;

1. *Affect the Mind*

Aphrodisiacs that affect the mind work by lowering inhibitions, which leads to impulses and sexual desires. Another way that they can affect the mind is by increasing the production of certain chemicals in the brain that are associated with sex and sexual arousal or desire.

2. *Affect the Body*

Aphrodisiacs that affect the bodywork by increasing blood flow to sexual areas of the body like the genitals or the nipples. This increase in blood flow causes feelings of sexual desire and arousal to arise for the person.

Examples of Aphrodisiacs

We will now look at some examples of aphrodisiacs so that you can get an idea of what foods and substances are included under this term.

Alcohol, Marijuana, and Drugs

To begin, we will look at two aphrodisiacs that you likely have heard of before. These are alcohol and marijuana. Marijuana and alcohol are both aphrodisiacs that work by lowering inhibitions in the mind. If you have ever been under the influence of either of these, you may have noticed that you felt more confident when it came to walking over to the bar to talk to that attractive person you had been eyeing, or that you were more forward in your sexual advances with your partner. This is because these substances lowered your inhibitions, which allowed your sexual impulses to take the driver's seat and motivated you to do things that you otherwise would not have due to the increased feelings of arousal that you were experiencing.

There are some other drugs that are known to lead to feelings of sexual arousal such as MDMA, and others that are known to actually lower libido such as some prescription drugs like antidepressants. The odd thing about alcohol as an aphrodisiac is that while it can lead to feelings of sexual arousal, it can also inhibit sexual performance, especially in males. There is a sweet spot here for increased sexual arousal before it becomes reduced performance.

Ginseng

Ginseng is an herb that is often found used in Chinese Medicine. It is often used to treat sexual dysfunction in both males and females, but it is quite strong and often reserved for males only. Ginseng can improve erectile dysfunction in men and can lead to greater levels of sexual arousal in women. It can be ingested in different ways, but the most common way in Asia is as a ginseng tea.

Pistachio

Pistachio nuts are proven to be an aphrodisiac. These nuts are found in a variety of dishes, both savory and sweet, and can be ingested whole. Pistachios have been shown to help with erectile dysfunction in men as it increases blood flow to the genitals. In women, this results in increased sexual arousal due to increased blood flow.

Other than being aphrodisiacs, pistachios boast many other health benefits, including blood pressure control, weight control, and improving heart function.

Saffron

Saffron is a spice that is used for a variety of purposes but is most often found in cooking derived from Southwest Asia. This spice is rare and quite expensive as it has to be harvested by hand and is very delicate.

At its origins, this spice has been used as a remedy for depression and mood disorders including stress reduction. Today, in men, it is an effective remedy for erectile dysfunction, and in women, it has been shown to increase sexual arousal and lubrication along with this. Saffron has been shown to be an effective aphrodisiac especially in people who are already taking antidepressants, as they often lead to reduced sexual drive and performance. If you are taking antidepressants and are experiencing a reduced sex drive, you will benefit from adding saffron into your diet if you have access to it.

Now we will move onto the fun ones, the aphrodisiacs that you have likely heard of before in the media or in conversation among friends.

Chocolate

Chocolate is an aphrodisiac that is fun to incorporate into your sex life, especially with a partner. Chocolate's aphrodisiac properties are due to the chemical compounds of cacao, which are proven to have aphrodisiac effects in women primarily.

Oysters

Oysters are a somewhat debated aphrodisiac but are commonly referred to as an aphrodisiac in the media. This could be more due to their texture, which reminds people of other erotic things and this leads to sexual thoughts and, therefore, sexual arousal. Either way, whether it is a placebo effect or not, its effects as an aphrodisiac have been reported in some people.

Honey

Honey's mention as an aphrodisiac, dates back centuries, as it was originally used ceremonially in marriages. Since then, it has been seen as a romantic food due to its texture and its silky appearance, which elicits sensual feelings in people. This puts them in the mood for sex and love.

Horny Goat Weed

You may have heard of this one before, but its actual name is Epimedium. This comes from Chinese Medicine as well and is often used here as a treatment for sexual dysfunction in men. It has also been shown to increase sexual arousal in women. Most of the uses and studies of these substances that have been used for centuries are focused on men and their effects on men, but many of them affect women just as well.

The name Horny Goat Weed comes from its effects on goats, which is, as legend has it, how it first became discovered as goats were found to act strangely after eating this specific weed. These days it can be ingested in pill form as a libido supporting supplement.

Chili Peppers

There is a compound within hot chili peppers that is called Capsaicin (which you have likely heard of). This is what makes chili peppers spicy. When spicy food is ingested, it leads to an increase in blood flow. In this specific case, capsaicin stimulates the nerve endings of the tongue, which then leads to the production and release of chemicals in the body that are known to increase sex drive and sexual arousal. If you notice that your tongue is on fire the next time you eat spicy food, you may find shortly after that you are feeling a little more aroused than you were before dinner.

How to Benefit from Them as a Couple

Now that you know what aphrodisiacs are and what some common examples of them are, we will now talk about how you can benefit from incorporating them into your sex life as a couple. There are numerous ways to use them and benefit from them.

Trouble Reaching Orgasm

The first way to benefit from the use of aphrodisiacs is either you or your partner experiences trouble reaching orgasm. This could be due to one of you taking antidepressants, experiencing high levels of stress, or a number of other reasons. If you or your partner are having trouble reaching orgasm, ingesting an aphrodisiac before having sex may help to give you that little something extra that you need to feel maximum pleasure. By eating something spicy for dinner or by drinking ginseng tea before having sex, this will help you to get into the mood and get your body ready for sex.

Pre- or During Sex Food Play

Another way that you can benefit from the use of aphrodisiacs as a couple is to make them part of your foreplay or your during-sex fun. This will help to make it feel less like ingesting an aphrodisiac clinically as an aid for sex and more as a sexy activity that you are doing together.

For example, incorporating chocolate covered strawberries or chocolate sauce into your foreplay by dripping it sexily over your partner's body and licking it off can help you to get aroused by its aphrodisiac effects and by the sensual and heat-building act of licking it off of each other's nipples. You can do the same with honey if you prefer it. Another way to do this is by having a pistachio or chocolate-filled dessert after dinner that you can feed each other while naked in order to get each other aroused and get your bodies ready for sex.

Menu Planning

By being aware of what aphrodisiacs you can incorporate into your sex life, you can use this with your partner in order to get creative together, designing the ideal menu for your dinner one day before having sex. You can make it fun by trying to develop the most delicious menu you can while trying to include the most aphrodisiacs you can in a single meal. You can include dessert in this plan, as well. Once you have come up with the menu, you can have fun shopping for all of these aphrodisiacs and cooking your meal together before eating it and then getting into bed together. This will make you both excited for the entire process from planning to shopping to cooking to eating and then having sex! Try this in order to connect in a variety of different ways over the course of the night, and this will lead to an increase in intimacy as well as an introduction of something new and fun into your sex life.

Aphrodisiacs are often joked about in conversation among friends and on the television. They are often not taken full advantage of in the sex lives of most people. After reading this chapter, you are fully informed so that you can begin to use these things to improve your sex life. Even if you are a skeptic, you can still have fun finding new ways to incorporate these with your partner. A placebo effect is an effect nonetheless!

Chapter 7
Sex Toys

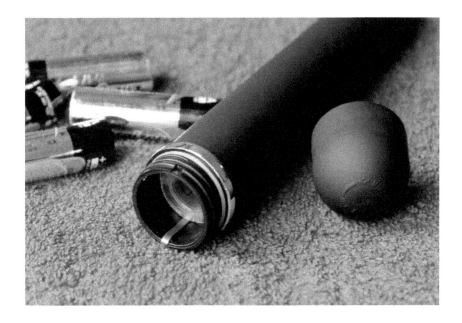

Sex toys may be something you are unfamiliar with, but they can bring fun, excitement, and new forms of pleasure to anybody's sex life. This chapter will help you to become aware of some of the sex toy options available to you and how they can be used to maximize both male and female pleasure. We will also look at how to use them safely and effectively and how to take advantage of all of their possibilities. additionally, in this chapter, we will look at everything related to sex toys and what they can offer you in your sex life with your partner as well as what you can do with them on your own. Remember, masturbation is a healthy part of anybody's sex life, even if they are in a long-term relationship. Sex toys are designed to increase and enhance pleasure; contrary to popular belief, they are not for people who need help sexually or who cannot perform on their own. The dialogue around sex toys and the fact that they are so taboo must be corrected if more people and couples want to unlock their full pleasure potential!

Sex Toys for Him

To begin, we are going to look at sex toys that men can benefit from as they are designed to be used with a penis. In this section, we are going to focus on how men can use and benefit from them on their own during masturbation, or how they can be used to please a man aside from penetration.

Cock Ring

The first sex toy we will look at is a cock ring. A cock ring was originally designed to keep a man's penis harder for a longer period of time. It does this because it is a ring made of metal that sits at the base of a man's penis, which helps to keep the blood flow inside of the penis for longer, which maintains an erection. These cock rings can be as tight or as loose as the man is comfortable with, as they come in a variety of sizes. This will also increase the man's pleasure as he will last longer.

Fleshlight

A fleshlight is another toy that is to be used by a man or anyone with a penis. This toy works by simulating a vagina or a mouth because of the way it looks and feels. Essentially it is a toy that can be disguised as a flashlight (which is how it got its name) because when it has the lid on, it looks very much like a flashlight. When you take off the lid, however, it looks like the opening of a vagina or mouth made of silicone. The man will insert his penis into the fleshlight and have penetrative sex with it as if it were a vagina or a mouth. The inside of the tube is texturized for added sensation. The soft silicone will feel similar to the skin of a woman, and this is why men find it a turn on to use this for masturbation rather than just their hand.

Sex doll

Similar to a fleshlight in some ways, is a sex doll. Instead of including only the vagina or the mouth like a fleshlight does, a sex doll is a doll that is modeled after the entire body of a woman, complete with holes in the mouth, the vagina, and sometimes the anus. It is used in a similar way as a fleshlight, where a man can insert his penis into any of these holes as if he were having sex with a woman.

The thing about a sex doll is that it is much less inconspicuous than a fleshlight or virtually any other sex toy as it is the size of a human when filled with air. It is similar to a pool toy, except that it is clearly used for sex. With this toy, it is very difficult to keep it out of sight from your partner, so keep this in mind when considering it.

Sex Toys For Her

Anything you can think of that would bring you sexual pleasure likely exists these days, and all it will take is a little bit of exploration to find out which toys you enjoy most. Don't be intimidated by all of the choices, as the purpose of all of this is to find pleasure! In this section, we are going to look at sex toys that women can benefit from as they are designed to be used with a clitoris or a vagina. In this section, we are going to focus on how women can use and benefit from these on their own during masturbation, or how they can be used to please her aside from penetration.

Vibrator

A vibrator is probably the most common sex toy available for female pleasure. Vibrators are the best choice for women who are new to sex toys and are unsure of what they may be looking for. A vibrator is a nice and easy place to start, and they can be used in a variety of ways. They are quite versatile in that they can be used by you alone, by you with a partner or by a partner to you during penetration or during foreplay. Vibrators come in so many different shapes, sizes, and materials.

Clitoral Vibrator

There are specific vibrators for the clitoris that are called clitoral vibrators that are small and compact, portable, and easy to use. This type of vibrator is turned on with the push of a button, and then you can hold it to your clitoris for quick and intense clitoral pleasure in a way like nothing else. Having something that is designed to be used on your clitoris that is also vibrating at speeds much higher than your hands could ever reach will be quite a new sensation, but one that you won't soon forget and will be quite eager to have again.

Bunny Ears Vibrator

There is another type of vibrator that is a little larger than a clitoral vibrator, and that also has an extra protruding piece on the side of it which can be inserted into the vagina so that you can have both vaginal penetration (so that you can stimulate your G-Spot) as well as vibrating, clitoral stimulation. This type is called a bunny ears vibrator since the portion that you insert into your vagina looks a little bit like bunny ears. With this shape, you can feel both of these types of pleasure at exactly the same time! This will be a new world of pleasure for you as you may never have had both your clitoris and your G-Spot stimulated at the same time.

This type of vibrator is usually made of silicone, and the small bump-like shape that juts out the side, which is the part that touches your clitoris, is also made of silicone. The entire vibrator will vibrate when you turn it on, so you will also feel some of the vibrations on your G-Spot as well, which will give you maximum pleasure.

Vibrating Dildo

The next type of vibrator we will look at is called a vibrating dildo. A dildo is a sex toy that is designed to be penis-like in shape, and that is usually made of silicone. A dildo is used by inserting it into either the vagina or the anus. This specific type of dildo is a sort of hybrid as it has the ability to act as a vibrator as well. This is usually done by way of a small bullet-shaped vibrator that is inserted into it. This type of vibrator allows you to have penetration with vibration. Because of this, the G-Spot can be stimulated and vibrated on at the same time, which will lead to intense pleasure.

This type of vibrator is good for someone who wants a more penis-like shape without specific clitoral stimulation, as some people prefer penetration over clitoral vibration. This type of dildo can also be worn as a strap-on, but we will visit that in the next section, so stay tuned.

Dildo

We already examined one specific type of dildo in the last section, but here we will look at the dildo as a sex toy on its own, without the vibrating option. If you are not a fan of the vibration and you don't need it, or if you simply don't want that function in your dildo, a regular dildo (like we will talk about here) is an option as well.

You have the option of using a more basic dildo that is simply a penis-like object that can come in a variety of different materials such as glass, stainless steel, or silicone. These can come in a wide variety of colors and shapes- from realistic-looking penises that come in a variety of skin tones, to pink and purple banana-shaped dildos. The world of dildos is vast and contains every and any kind of penetrative device you could possibly dream of.

Dildos can be used by a woman alone while masturbating by being inserted into the vagina in order to stimulate her G-Spot. While doing this, you can also massage your clitoris with your other hand, or you can stick with the vaginal stimulation on its own. Most dildos can be taken into the bathtub or shower as well, as they are all waterproof (except the vibrating kind) so you can have shower sex with your dildo if you wish.

A dildo can be used in the vagina or the anus, whichever you prefer, and you can use the same dildo for both of these places, so you don't need to buy two. If you want to use your dildo during a solo session, you can insert it into your anus in a similar way as you would insert it into your vagina. Just be sure that when switching between the anus and the vagina, you thoroughly clean the dildo and/or your hands to prevent the chance of an infection. You could also insert the dildo into your vagina while you massage or penetrate your anus using your hand. You can really do anything you like with a dildo, any combination of sexual acts that turn you on and get you to orgasm.

Sex Toys for Him or Her

Following our discussion of sex toys for men and for women, we will now look at some toys that can be used by both men and women, either during a solo pleasure session or by a partner.

Nipple Clamps

The next sex toy we will look at are nipple clamps. Nipple clamps are usually made of silver or another metal of some sort and are clipped onto the nipples, which pinches them. The two clamps are often connected by a chain, and this causes the clamps to pull down on the nipples for added sensation.

This sex toy falls loosely into the category of sadism and masochism, which is a category within BDSM since there is a low level of pain involved in this. The level of pain can be controlled or adjusted, depending on how sensitive your nipples are and how much pain you enjoy to become turned on during sex. If you enjoy a higher level of pain, you can get nipple clamps of a heavier weight, and if you only want a little bit (especially if you have very sensitive nipples), you can get lighter ones. This depends on the type of metal they are made of, the thickness of the clamps, and the weight of the chain that connects them. If you enjoy the pinching of the clamps on your nipples because it stimulates them and makes you aroused, but you prefer not to have the chain pulling them down too aggressively, then you can opt for the light chain and clamps.

While wearing nipple clamps, you are free to touch and stimulate every other part of your own body while you experience the pleasure from the stimulation of your nipples. This is the benefit of nipple clamps as it allows for hands-off pleasure, so you are free to focus on other parts of your body.

When using these with a partner, you and your partner are both free to stimulate every part of each other's bodies, as neither of you will have to stimulate each other's or their own nipples because the clamps take care of that for you. Then, you are both free to touch each other's genitals. The only difference that may be noted between men and women when using nipple clamps is that the weight desired by men and women to achieve pleasurable pain could be different- a man may want heavier ones compared to a woman.

Anal Toys

Following our brief discussion of the possibilities of anal pleasure with a dildo in an earlier section within this chapter, we will now look at some more specific toys for anal pleasure. There are a variety of anal toys that you can use to give yourself pleasure, either actively or passively.

Butt Plug

The butt plug is a toy that is used passively to give you pleasure anally while you are busy doing other things with your hands. A butt plug is a small silicone or glass device that is inserted into the anus and is left there. This provides pleasure from the stretching of the anal opening, which, as I mentioned, is very sensitive. It also provides pleasure from the stretching of the anal canal in general, and as you move, you will feel pleasure from the pressure it puts on the inside of your anus. This type of anal toy can be used in preparation for anal sex in order to encourage the anal canal to relax, or to get a head start on pleasure during foreplay or before sex entirely. Either a woman or a man can use a butt plug during a solo session by inserting it and leaving it inserted while massaging their clitoris, using another sex toy vaginally, or (for a man) stimulating their penis. This way it can provide passive pleasure during other acts.

Anal Beads

Another anal toy that can be used for great pleasure are anal beads. Anal beads are a series of beads, arranged in order of size starting from smallest to largest, that are all attached together and that have a ring at the end, closest to the largest bead. These can be inserted into the anus all the way until just the ring is exposed at the end. What this does is allow you to insert the bigger beads last since you first inserted smaller ones, which gradually increased in size, preparing your anus for the larger sized ones. When they are inside of you, it will work similarly to a butt plug in that it will give your anus pleasurable internal pressure, as well as pleasure from the stretching of the sensitive anal opening, especially as the beads increase in size. This type of anal sex toy is an active type as it is used by being moved, providing active pleasure.

How Couples Can Use Sex Toys Together

Sex toys may be a new area of exploration for a lot of couples when in the bedroom together, even if the two people have experience with sex toys on their own. Many sex toys that can be used solo can also be used as a couple. With the advent of so many new technologies in this day and age, the potential is endless.

Using a Cock Ring as a Couple

A cock ring has another use than just for a man during masturbation. A cock ring can be used as a couple together during penetrative sex, as well. The first benefit of using a cock ring as a couple is that because it keeps a man's penis erect for much longer, the woman will be able to experience more pleasure due to a longer period during which penetration can happen. This effect will help her to orgasm from penetration because, as you now know, a woman requires a continued and prolonged stimulation of her G-Spot in order to reach orgasm.

Another benefit of using a cock ring as a couple is that there is another type of cock ring which has vibrating functions. A cock ring like this works in much the same way as the metal ones but is usually made of a softer material like silicone, and it begins vibrating with the push of a button or the flip of a switch. While the man is wearing this, it will vibrate on the base of his penis, which will be pleasurable for him and keep him erect for longer, but it will also act as a vibrator on the woman's clitoris during penetration.

Using a Dildo or Strap-On as a Couple

Dildos can be used with a partner as well as used solo by a woman, as we have seen. If a woman enjoys the feeling of being penetrated by a dildo, her partner can hold it and insert it into her vagina while she lies back and enjoys the sensation, or while she stimulates her own clitoris at the same time.

A dildo can also be used as a couple for something called Pegging. Many heterosexual couples practice Pegging, or anal sex from a woman to a man using a sex toy, usually a dildo. When a dildo is inserted into a harness that is worn by a woman around her legs and waist, it is called a strap-on. Any type of dildo can be inserted into a harness to become a strap-on. Pegging is done to stimulate a man anally when his partner is holding a dildo or wearing it as a strap-on. The pleasure potential of a man's anus is usually only discussed in relation to homosexual males, but anal pleasure is not only reserved for gay couples and should be fully explored by any man or heterosexual couple wanting to unlock the full pleasure that a man's body is capable of.

There is another kind of dildo that is used to achieve both male and female pleasure at the same time. This is a Double-Ended Dildo. This type is not worn as a strap-on but is instead used by being inserted into the man's anus while also being inserted into either the woman's anus or her vagina. Then, both people can thrust towards each other to pleasure each other at the same time. This type of dildo has the ability to please the woman in multiple ways and also has the ability to please the man to a great degree. While being penetrated in this way, the woman can also use a vibrator or another type of sex toy to stimulate her clitoris if she wishes.

Using Anal Toys as a Couple

As we previously discussed, anal toys can be used by either men or women to experience pleasure. In this section, we will look at how they can be used together as a couple.

A butt plug can be used as a couple by being left in place while having penetrative sex by either the man or woman or both. To use this as a couple, you can insert them for each other and then leave them inserted while you begin penetration. This will lead to great pleasure, especially for the woman as the pressure the butt plug places on the inside of the anal walls, in combination with the pressure that the man's penis puts on the inside of the vaginal walls come together to stimulate both the anus and the vagina at the exact same time. Also, because both of these canals have something filling them, there is an increase in the general pressure of the entire genital area, which will lead to high levels of overall pleasure for the woman. This increase in pressure of the vagina will also be felt by the penis of the man since he is inserting his penis into a smaller canal. The thrusting in and out by the man's penis while a butt plug is inserted will cause the woman and the man to feel varying levels of pressure.

A woman may be able to have a blended anal and a vaginal orgasm in this way, and if she is looking for even more pleasure, she or her partner can also massage or use a vibrator on her clitoris to stimulate all three areas at once. This will create the potential of three distinct and blended orgasms.

Chapter 8
Sex Positions

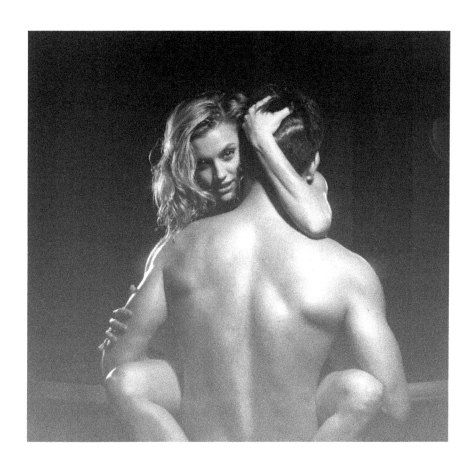

As your relationship progresses, it is important to keep sex and lust alive. When you become progressively more and more comfortable with someone, it can take away some of the mystery. This is because there is no longer the excitement of getting to know a person, and having everything you do together be brand new. Getting to this point in your relationship is fun and comforting in its own way, and is different from, but in some ways better than, the early stages. From a sexual perspective, though, we don't want the coming of this stage of your relationship to bring with it the end of an exciting sex life. This next chapter will teach you how to maintain the lust and intimacy and keep welcoming new sexual adventures together as an established couple.

Sensual Positions for Maximum Intimacy

Intimacy is something that needs to be worked at and practiced. It is something that needs to be actively maintained and does not stay as-is when achieved once. As a couple, there are many ways to work on your intimacy, and sex is one of those ways. Sex also happens to come with many other benefits, but these positions we will explore now are chosen because they are the best for creating intimacy and connection for you and your partner.

The Lotus

Arguably the most intimate position of them all is The Lotus. The Lotus position is most intimate because of the closeness of your entire bodies, infinitely pressed against each other at all points from head to toe while being face to face.

The man sits on the bed cross-legged, his torso upright. His penis is erect and ready to get it on. The woman climbs on top of him and sits in his lap, wrapping her arms and legs around him. He holds her by wrapping his arms around her as well. With some shifting, they slide his penis inside of her. In this position, both people will be grinding more than they will be thrusting or humping. This is also what makes it so intimate. Grinding face to face while she is sitting on his lap with him inside of her, that is about as intimate as it gets.

In this position, you will not be doing any crazy thrusting, so it is ideal for a steamy make-out session, as your mouths will be so close that you can feel each other's breath the entire time. You can look into each other's eyes and whisper sweet nothings to them as you share this intimate experience.

Slow Grind

Another position that makes for a high level of intimacy and closeness is the Slow Grind position. In this position, the man sits down with his legs extended and leans back on his hands. The woman climbs on top of him, facing him and puts his penis inside of her. she extends her legs past him and leans back on her hands as well. In this position, they cannot move too much without risking his penis sliding out of her, so they are restricted to a slow grind. They both slowly grind their hips into each other and move gently. With both of their arms occupied to hold them up, they can only move their hips, and this makes for an intimate mood with no distractions of arms and legs moving about. They are seated facing each other as well, so they will look at each other in the eyes as they slowly grind and pleasure each other. You can see why this position is such an intimate one for a couple to try together.

Spicy Positions for More Adventure

If you are a long-term or married couple, you have likely tried every one of the classic sex positions together from missionary to 69. You have probably also developed a routine of your favorite positions and the order in which you do them by now. While you probably know how to please each other like it's second nature, rediscovering each other's bodies in a sexy way and learning new ways to pleasure each other is good for couples who have been together for a long time.

Reverse Cowgirl with Anal Play

This position is a new take on an old classic. Get into the reverse cowgirl position, which means that the man lies down on the bed on his back, and the woman straddles his penis; however, she is facing his feet instead of his head. From this position, the woman can grind her hips on the man's penis and control the speed and depth of penetration. To make it an advanced position; however, she will lean forward and can grab onto his ankles for support. Then, he can begin to play with her anus using his fingers or a toy. He does not need to penetrate her there; necessarily, he can just play with the outside of her anus, and she will still feel immense amounts of pleasure.

The Waterfall

The waterfall is a position that can bring something new to your bedroom routine. This position requires some flexibility and strength from both people but holds lots of pleasure potential.

The man will begin by sitting in a chair with his feet on the floor. The woman will climb onto his lap and insert his penis into her. She can wrap her legs around his waist. Then, slowly, she will lean all the way back until her head and arms are touching the floor (with pillows underneath). From here, the man will hold onto her hips and can move her body onto his penis at whatever speed and depth he wishes. He can also grab onto her breasts and massage her clitoris in this position if he wishes.

Chapter 9
Kama Sutra: Tantric Positions for His Pleasure

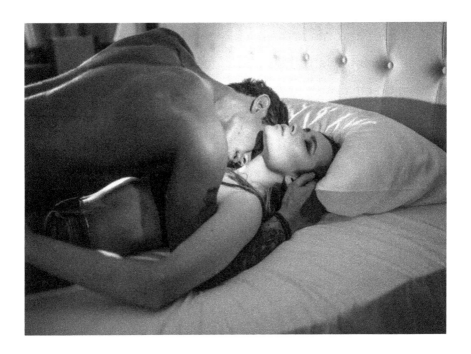

The Mare's Position

This position is a position that comes from The Kama Sutra. This position is great for the man's pleasure because of the technique it involves on the part of the woman, more than the position itself. This technique has the potential to change your sexual life forever.

In this position, the man sits with his legs stretched out in front of him and his arms back, supporting his weight on the bed. The woman straddles him, facing away from him and lowers herself down onto his erect penis. Once his penis is inside of her, the woman uses her vaginal muscles to apply and release pressure on the man's penis, almost as if she is milking it. This is how it got its name. This technique makes for very pleasurable sensations on the man's penis as it creates varying pressure while he is penetrating her. It creates more stimulation on the man's penis than just classic penetration. As a bonus, this also strengthens the woman's vaginal muscles, which in time will lead to stronger orgasms for her.

Tripod Position

This position is one where the woman and man are both standing. The woman and man will both stand facing each other and the man will hold onto one of the woman's legs under her knee. The man will hold her leg raised and enter her from beneath. Because there are only three legs on the ground, this is called the Tripod Position. This position allows for maximum blood flow to the genitals, leading to great male pleasure.

Piditaka Position

This position is another Kama Sutra position, that requires some flexibility but is relaxing once you get into it. The woman lies back on the bed and lifts her knees, putting them on the man's chest. The man will get on top of the woman and holds her knees against his chest. The man will put his knees on either side of her buttocks and enter her from this position. This position is good for male pleasure as the vagina is narrowed while the woman's legs are up, which feels great on his penis.

Hanging position

This position is similar to the standing position, but it is different in that it involves a little more support. The man will stand up with his back against a wall, with the woman standing and facing him. The woman will jump into the man's arms and he will hold her up by her buttocks. The woman will extend her legs behind her and rest them on the wall. This position feels great for the man since the woman's vagina is closed up and this makes a tighter environment for the penis.

The Bent Position

The woman will lie down on the floor and lift her legs up, bringing her knees to her chest and widening them. She will hold onto her legs under her knees to keep them lifted. The man will crouch low in a squat position and lean forward to enter the woman from below. He can hold onto her legs for support as he thrusts into her. Since the woman's legs are lifted, this position feels great on the man's penis.

The Cow Position

The Cow Position is a position where the man will enter the woman from behind. The woman will lie face down on a bed with a pillow underneath her hips to lift her buttocks off the bed a bit. The man will get on top of the woman and enter her. This position is good for male pleasure since it provides him with the opportunity to control the pace and the depth.

Fixing A Nail

The woman will lie on her back and the man comes over top of her and lifts one of her legs. He will lift her leg so that her foot is planted on his forehead. He can then enter her from the front while keeping her foot on his head. As he thrusts into her, she will alternate her feet on his head and this will change the feelings for each of them, providing them with variety.

The Peg

The man lies on his side and the woman lies facing him on her side, with her head towards his feet. The woman will lift her knees towards her chest and place one of her legs underneath the man's legs and have the other on top of his legs. Essentially, she is hugging his legs with her entire body. She slides up so that her vulva is next to his penis. When aligned properly he can penetrate her and can achieve depth and control as she is positioned perfectly for his penis to enter her. The woman wraps her arms around his legs and he can use his hands and arms to help with his thrusting.

Chapter 10
Kama Sutra: Tantric Positions for Her Pleasure

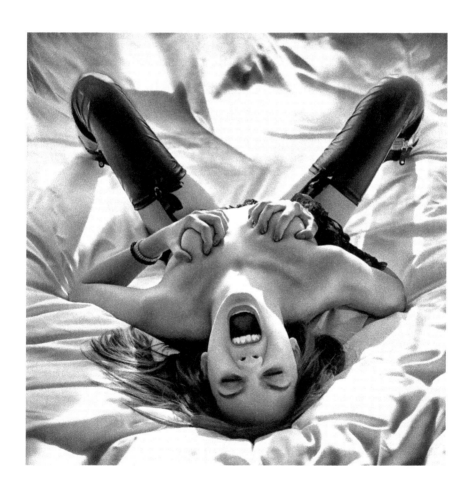

These positions that follow are best for the female orgasm and the pleasure of the woman. For great pleasure for the woman, positions that maximize G-Spot contact, as well as positions that allow for simultaneous clitoral stimulation, are best.

Standing Suspended

This first position is a position that comes from the Kama Sutra. This position is great for the female orgasm because of the angle that the man's penis enters her vagina and also because the man is in control in this position so the woman can relax and enjoy the pleasure he is bringing to her body.

To get into this position, the man will stand facing a wall with the woman standing in front of him, her back to the wall. She will then jump into his arms and wrap both her arms and her legs around him. Once here, he can insert his penis into her vagina while holding onto her buttocks or underneath her knees. He can lean her back on the wall in front of him for support so that he does not have to support her entire weight in his arms. If he holds onto her underneath her knees, this will open her up so that her vagina is easily accessible. The fact that she is suspended coupled with this will make it so that there is deep penetration occurring, and this will be pleasurable for both the man and the woman. Deep penetration is great for the female orgasm because there are two places located deep within the vagina that, when stimulated, lead to a very intense orgasm for her. The penis must achieve continuous deep penetration in order for this to happen and in this position, it is quite possible.

The Peasant

This position is great for the woman as she will receive clitoral stimulation as well as penetration. To get into this position, the man will sit on the floor or the bed and the woman will sit on top of his lap. The woman will spread her legs wide and the man will insert his penis into her from behind. The man will reach around her and stimulate her clitoris while the woman grinds on his lap.

The Rider Position

The man will lie on his back and lift his knees to his chest, spreading them wide. The woman will then sit on the man, underneath his bent legs and sit on his penis. She can hold on his bent knees for support, and grind on his penis or lift her body up and down on him. This position is great for female pleasure since she can touch her clitoris or the man can stimulate it for her. It is also pleasurable for her as she can control the movement.

Indrani

This position is more acrobatic than many other Kama Sutra positions. The woman will lie on her back and the man will kneel in front of her, near her legs. The man will lift her up by the buttocks and put his penis into her. He will hold onto her thighs to keep her buttocks lifted off of the bed. This position leads to interruptions an changes in blood flow, which will make the woman feel immense pleasure.

Milk And Water Embrace

This position is sensual and romantic, while also allowing for clitoral stimulation. The man will sit in a chair and the woman will sit on his lap, facing away from him. The woman and man will both grind their hips into each other and the man can reach his hand around and stimulate her clitoris.

The Yawning Position

The woman lies on her back and spreads her legs out as wide as she can. The man will enter the woman from the front with his knees underneath her hips. He can lean forward and their faces can come close together int his position.

The Rocking Horse

This position is a woman on top position. This makes it easier for her to feel pleasure since the angle of the man's penis inside of her will hit her G-Spot. The man sits down on the floor with his arms outstretched behind him. The woman will straddle the man, facing him. She will hug his thighs with hers and move her hips to control the thrusting. Since they are both sitting up, this position makes for a tight embrace.

The Cross

The woman lies on her back with one leg extended straight into the air. The man kneels in front of her, straddling her leg that is extended on the bed and holds onto her other leg which is in the air. He can then move his body forward between her two legs until he is close enough to insert his penis into her vagina. He can hold her legs spread with his body, straddling one of them and placing the other one on his shoulder. By doing this, his hands will be free so that he can play with her clitoris, massage her breasts, rubbing his hands up and down her body or whatever they please.

The Yab-Yum Position

To continue our exploration of Tantric Sex, this next position is a very versatile and introductory position that beginners and masters alike use daily in their practices. This staple position of Tantric Sex is called the Yab-Yum position. You can do this position with clothes on or without. You can use it in a non-sexual moment of connection with your partner, you can use it get into the mood for sex, or you can use it as a position during sexual intercourse itself.

You can do this position anywhere, whether on a bed or on the floor, whatever is most comfortable. First, one partner sits cross-legged, and then the other partner sits in their lap, facing them, with their legs wrapped around their partner's waist. From this face to face position you can see deep into your partner's eyes, you can feel their breath as their chest rises and falls, and you can feel and sense all of the small movements and sensations of their body that you would not otherwise perceive. Get quiet in this position together to start. Just sit and experience this closeness, take in everything with each other and let the moment evolve; however, it does. Let it lead to whatever it leads to. Maybe beginning this position fully clothed and with the intention of just connecting spiritually will lead to such an intense moment of connection that you will rip each other's clothes off and have the best orgasms you have ever had because of this connection. Maybe you stay in this position with clothes on, and you feel closer emotionally. Either one is perfect.

If you want to do this position solely for the purpose of

penetration, try beginning by syncing your breathing together before starting to get really into the humping and the coming. This will make the position somewhat Tantric, at least, and will lead to more satisfying orgasms. When getting into this position for the purpose of sex only, begin already naked with your partner and get into the position as explained above, but make sure to have the man on the bottom and the woman on top. The woman, as the top, will need to adjust her hips in order to align your genitals with hers to allow for penetration. Once the penis is inside of the vagina, you will be linked in this tight, extremely close position. Now you can begin to thrust and grind and grope and everything else that pushes you both over the edge.

Chapter 11
How to Last Longer

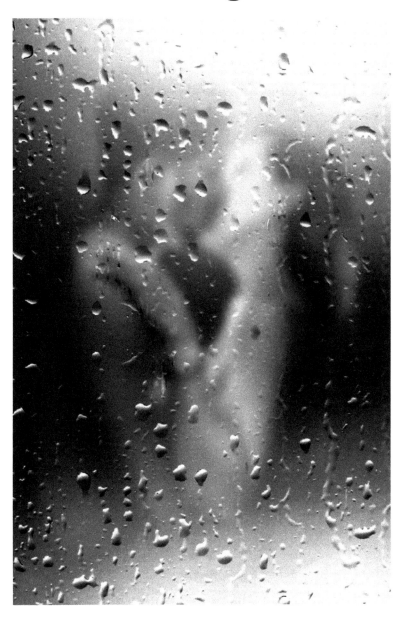

There are many theories regarding how to last longer and how to stay harder, and we will look at a few of the most effective ones now in this section. In order for both men and women to get the most out of sex and the most enjoyable orgasms, it comes down to the man's ability to last during sex. If the time it takes a man to orgasm is quite short, then the pair will have to wait until his refractory period is over before he will be able to have an erection again. During this time, the woman will still be able to be aroused and have an orgasm, but penetrative sex will not be possible. Thus, in order to have the most pleasurable and (and also more intense) orgasms and sexual encounters, I will now present some tips and tricks that the man can use to last longer in bed.

Edging

Edging is a technique that a man can use to hold off an orgasm to make himself last longer and therefore keep his erection for longer. In order to do this, he must be aware of his body and be in touch with the different feelings it has. This is similar to what we discussed earlier when talking about mindfulness and how it relates to sex.

When the man reaches a point where he is getting very close to orgasm, he will stop, or the woman will stop whatever they are doing, and he will have to take a deep breath, compose himself and hold off his orgasm. Holding back will give him time to cool down a little and come back from the edge of orgasm. During this time, while he is cooling off, he can continue to touch the woman, or the woman can touch him in other places, as long as it doesn't make him orgasm. When he is ready and has successfully held off his orgasm, they can then continue with whatever sexual acts they were doing before. Then, when he reaches the point where he is about to orgasm again, he will have to hold off once again. This can continue as many times as he can until finally one time, he will let himself reach orgasm, and it will be much stronger and much more intense than if he had just let himself reach orgasm the first time.

This may be difficult to accomplish the first number of times because it can be hard to hold off an orgasm when you are very close. It will take practice to be able to do this technique, and especially to be able to do it multiple times over in one session. The man will have to communicate with his partner so that she knows not to keep stimulating him to the point of orgasm, especially if she was giving him oral or something of the sort.

Going to the Gym

Another way that a man can increase his endurance sexually is by going to the gym. Physical fitness is strongly related to sexual performance and endurance, so getting to the gym at least a few times a week will help him to last longer in bed, keep his erection longer and even to be able to thrust for longer because of the cardiovascular aspect that penetrative sex comes with. This will be beneficial for both of you.

Chapter 12
Beyond the Bedroom

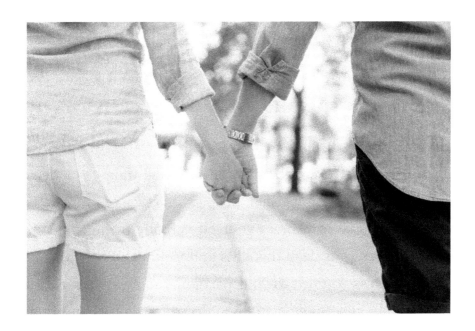

As a long-term couple, it is important that you remain intimate with each other not only in the bedroom, but outside of it as well. Since a relationship is about much more than the sex, your emotional intimacy is a large part of what keeps you together. As we discussed at the beginning of this book, there are different forms of intimacy. Until now, we have focused on physical or sexual intimacy, but now we are going to switch over and focus on the other types.

Emotional Intimacy

Just to remind you, emotional intimacy is the ability to express oneself in a mature and open manner, leading to a deep emotional connection between people. This type of intimacy is about being able to express yourself verbally using language that describes your deep thoughts and feelings. When you are able to express yourself to your partner, you create a sense of understanding between you that deepens your connection. When both of you are able to do this, you will maintain that deep connection between you. Intimacy must also be maintained, and this is done by ensuring that you are continuing to express your deep thoughts and feelings with your partner, even when you become very comfortable with them. When you reach a point where you feel like you know each other so well that you can read each other like a book, it is still important to be open verbally with your partner to keep the lines of communication open.

Expressing yourself verbally can be done by saying things like "I love you" or "thank you for being there for me." When you do this, you are reminding your partner how you feel and that you appreciate them. This is important to say, even if you know that they know how you feel. It is still nice for them to hear it from you. This creates deeper emotional intimacy. This can also be done by expressing yourself in terms of other things like why you had a bad day, what you are nervous about or what you want to share with them. Having a person close to you of this sort allows you to have someone to express yourself to, and they can express themselves to you. By doing this, you not only are able to express yourself in a healthy way, but you also are maintaining the relationship in a deep way.

Intimacy Beyond The Bedroom

There are some ways that you can maintain a good level of emotional intimacy with your partner, in order to ensure that you remain connected and in love for as long as possible. Below, I have outlined some of these ways.

Spend Time

The first way is to spend time with your partner doing things that both of you find enjoyable that you can share. When you spend quality time together, even if you are not doing anything extremely exciting, having time to simply talk and connect will help you to maintain your connection with each other and continue to know each other on and keep level as you both change and grow.

Be Curious

This brings us to our next point, which is to stay curious. Remaining curious in your relationship is one of the most important things you can do. By remaining curious about your partner and making an effort to get to know them over and over again, you will keep your relationship interesting, and you will keep knowing your partner even as they may change. This goes for every part of them, from their likes and dislikes about food, in bed, with television shows and so on.

You also want to remain curious about your relationship. By remaining curious about your relationship, you can consistently ensure that you will be giving your all and making it the best relationship it can be. Remain curious about what you can do better and what is working well in your relationship with your partner.

As you continue on in your relationship with your partner, you never know when the knowledge this book has bestowed on, you will prove useful. You may want to try something new on an anniversary getaway and think of the perfect position to try (from chapter 9 or 10), you may be having a discussion with your friends about marriage and sex and you may think of how you learned that intimacy must be maintained and worked at (chapter 1) in order to remain strong. This knowledge will remain in the back of your mind until the time when you need it most, and then it will pop to the front of your mind in order to help yourself, your partner, or your friends. You can never be too knowledgeable about sex and relationships, and by taking the step to read this book in its entirety, you are only helping yourself out for the rest of your life- your sex life, your romantic life, and your life in general.

Conclusion

Thank you for reaching the end of this book. I hope that you have learned a lot about yourself and your sex life and how you can improve your sex life with your partner. It may seem like a lot to take in and process, but as you let this information sink in, it will become clearer to you.

How to Apply What You Have Learned

After reading this book, it is now in your hands to apply what you have learned. In this section, I will provide you with some tips for how you can begin to incorporate this into your life in general as well as your sex life.

The first tip I will share is to begin slowly and deliberately. You do not need to force yourself to begin applying everything covered into this book into your life, as it will likely overwhelm you and your partner, and this could lead to more stress than anything else. Begin by picking out one or two things that you would like to begin with. For example, Tantric Massage and longer foreplay. These two will go together well as during foreplay is a great time to practice Tantra. You can begin by explaining to your partner what exactly it is, what it entails, and how you want them to support you in this new endeavor.

You can then begin by taking the lead and practicing tantric breathing and massage together. After this, once you are fully in the moment and feeling your pleasure as well as each other's energy, you can keep going with your foreplay for as long as you like.

Remember to remain patient, as it may take some time to become comfortable and familiar with these new practices or techniques, especially if your partner has not read this book for themselves. By being patient with yourself and your partner, you will be able to look at the incorporation of these new techniques and practices as a gradual exploration that you are doing together rather than something that must be conquered and mastered in one session.

Communication

As you know, by this point in the book, I am a strong believer that communication is the key to everything. To solving problems, to strengthening any type of relationship, and to moving past rough spots. Sex is no different, and communication will make your sex life as comfortable and enjoyable as it can possibly be.

By sharing this book with your partner, you will be able to communicate about it afterward. This will help to open up a dialogue about sex, which is especially beneficial if you have had a hard time opening dialogue about this topic in the past. You can discuss the parts you liked about the book, the parts you disliked, and the parts that left you with questions. You can address these together, and this can often lead to a discussion about sex in general. This is the time that you can then ask your partner if they feel like there is anything missing from your sex life, if there is anything they love about it or if there is anything they would like to change. This can also be a time for you to open up about your thoughts and feelings regarding this. This leads to our discussion of emotional intimacy, as this type of communication will lead to a deeper connection between the two of you.

Take this book and the information contained in it forward with you into whatever presents itself next in your life. If you enjoyed it, share it with your friends, and they will be thanking you for bettering their relationships and their sex lives for years to come.